Social Theory and Nursing Practice

D1078293

WITHDRAWN FROM STOCK

Sociology and Nursing Practice Series

Margaret Miers
Gender Issues and Nursing Practice

Sam Porter
Social Theory and Nursing Practice

Geoff Wilkinson (editor)
Power and Nursing Practice

Sociology and Nursing Practice Series
Series Standing Order
ISBN 0–333–69329–9
(outside North America only)

You can receive future titles in this series as they are published by placing a standing o
Please contact your bookseller or, in the case of difficulty, write to us at the address be
with your name and address, the title of the series and the ISBN quoted above.

Customer Services Department, Macmillan Distribution Ltd
Houndmills, Basingstoke, Hampshire RG21 6XS, England

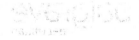

Social Theory and Nursing Practice

Sam Porter

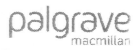

5155321.

© Sam Porter 1998

Series Preface © Margaret Miers, Sam Porter and Geoff Wilkinson 1998

All rights reserved. No reproduction, copy or transmission of this
publication may be made without written permission.

No paragraph of this publication may be reproduced, copied or transmitted
save with written permission or in accordance with the provisions of the
Copyright, Designs and Patents Act 1988, or under the terms of any licence
permitting limited copying issued by the Copyright Licensing Agency, 90
Tottenham Court Road, London W1T 4LP.

Any person who does any unauthorised act in relation to this publication
may be liable to criminal prosecution and civil claims for damages.

The author has asserted his right to be identified as the author of this work
in accordance with the Copyright, Designs and Patents Act 1988.

First published 1998 by
PALGRAVE MACMILLAN
Houndmills, Basingstoke, Hampshire RG21 6XS and
175 Fifth Avenue, New York, N.Y. 10010
Companies and representatives throughout the world

PALGRAVE MACMILLAN is the global academic imprint of the Palgrave
Macmillan division of St. Martin's Press, LLC and of Palgrave Macmillan Ltd.
Macmillan® is a registered trademark in the United States, United Kingdom
and other countries. Palgrave is a registered trademark in the European
Union and other countries.

ISBN-13: 978–0–333–69197-7paperback
ISBN-10: 0–333–69197-0 paperback

This book is printed on paper suitable for recycling and made from fully
managed and sustained forest sources. Logging, pulping and manufacturing
processes are expected to conform to the environmental regulations of the
country of origin

A catalogue record for this book is available from the British Library.

Printed and bound in Great Britain by
Biddles Ltd., King's Lynn, Norfolk

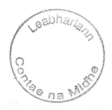

Do Siobhán agus Ewan
Bualtrai arís

Contents

Series Editors' Preface   x
Acknowledgements   xii

1 **Introduction**   1
   The structure of the book   5
   The structure of chapters   6
   Sic men   6

PART I **Getting to the roots**   9

2 **Structural functionalism and role theory**   11
   Introduction   11
   The Hobbesian problem of order   13
   Durkheim and social solidarity   14
   Anomic suicide   17
   The pertinence of Durkheim to nursing   22
   Parsons' structural functionalism   22
   The pattern variables of the medical role   26
   Nursing example: gender and professional roles   27
   The sick role   31
   Nursing example: the unpopular patient   32
   Assessing Parsons' role theory   33
   Recommended further reading   33

3 **Marxism and the political economy of health**   34
   Introduction   34
   Karl Marx   34
   Historical materialism   35
   Marxist explanations of ill health   40
   Exploitation and illness   42
   Capitalism and health care   45
   Making profits from illness   52
   Nursing example: Marxism and informal care   54
   Recommended further reading   57

4 **Weber and professional closure**   58
   Introduction   58
   Class, status and party   59

Education and social closure   63
The social closure of professions   64
Dual closure strategies   69
Gender and professions   71
Nursing example: registration and dual closure   72
Nursing example: the limits of social closure   77
The Marxist reposte   80
Recommended further reading   82

PART II Getting to the action   83

5   Symbolic interactionism, labelling and stigma   85
    Introduction   85
    George Herbert Mead's social psychology   86
    Herbert Blumer's definition   87
    Labelling theory   90
    Mental illness as labelled deviance   91
    Total institutions   92
    Stigma   95
    Nursing example: nurses' power in interactions
    with patients   100
    Recommended further reading   103

6   Phenomenology and ethnomethodology   105
    Introduction   105
    Husserl and phenomenology   105
    Weber and *Verstehen*   109
    Schutz and phenomenological sociology   111
    Nursing example: the phenomenology of comfort 114
    Ethnomethodology   117
    Nursing example: the ethnomethodology of home
    visiting   122
    Recommended further reading   124

PART III Bringing it all together   125

7   Critical theory and communicative action   129
    Introduction   129
    The roots of critical theory   129
    The Frankfurt school   132
    The influence of phenomenology   136
    Habermas and communicative action   138
    Weber's theory of rationality   139
    Habermas on rationality   141
    The purposive rationality of medicine   146

Nursing example: new nursing as communicative action   149
Recommended further reading   152

8   Structuration theory and critical realism   154
Introduction   154
Giddens' critiques of interpretative and structural theories   155
Structuration theory   160
Nursing example: the intrusion of the social   164
Archer's critique of structuration theory   167
Bhaskar and critical realism   171
Nursing example: racism and professionalism   175
Conclusion   178
Recommended further reading   178

PART IV   Taking it all apart   179

9   Feminisms, caring and women's knowledge   181
Introduction   181
The development of feminist approaches   181
Cultural feminism   189
The ethic of care   189
Nursing example: women and AIDS   192
Feminist epistemology   194
Standpoint feminism   196
Nursing example: nursing knowledge, women's
knowledge   200
The significance of accepting difference   202
Recommended further reading   203

10   Postmodernism and Foucault   204
Introduction   204
Modernism   204
Postmodernism   206
Foucault and knowledge   209
Nursing example: nursing as textually mediated discourse   213
Foucault and power   216
Nursing example: the surveillance of health visitors   222
Conclusion   224
Recommended further reading   225

Afterword   227

References   230

Name index   240

Subject index

Series Editors' Preface

It is widely accepted that because sociology can provide nurses with valuable and pertinent insights, it should be a constituent part of nursing's knowledge base. To take but a few substantive examples, sociology can help nurses to understand the causes and distribution of ill health, the experience of illness, the dynamics of health care encounters and the limitations and possibilities of professional care. Equally importantly, sociology's emphasis on critical reflection can encourage nurses to be more questioning and self-aware, thus helping them to provide flexible, non-discriminatory, client-centred care.

Unfortunately, while the aspiration of integrating sociology into nursing knowledge is easy enough to state in theory, in practice their relationship has not been as productive as some might have hoped. Notwithstanding a number of works that have successfully applied sociological tools to nursing problems, there remains a gulf between the two disciplines, which has led some to question the utility of the relationship.

On the one hand, sociologists, while taking an interest in nursing's occupational position, have not paid great attention to the actual work that nurses do. This is partially the result of the limitations of sociological surveillance. Nurses work in confidential, private and intimate settings with their clients, and sociologists' access to such settings is necessarily restricted. Moreover, nurses find it difficult to talk about their work, except to other nurses. As a result, core issues pertaining to nursing have been less than thoroughly treated in the sociological literature. There is thus a disjunction between what nurses require from sociology and what sociologists can provide.

On the other hand, nurses are on equally uncertain ground when they attempt to use sociology themselves. Nurses are often reliant on carefully simplified introductory texts, which, because of their broad remit, are often unable to provide an in-depth understanding of sociological insights. Nor is it simply a matter of knowledge; there are tensions between the outlooks of nursing and of sociology. Because nursing work involves individual inter-actions, it is not surprising that when nurses turn to sociology, they turn to those elements that concentrate on microsocial inter-action. While this is useful in so far as it goes, it does not provide nurses with knowledge of the restraints and enablements imposed upon individual actions by social structures.

The aim of the *Sociology and Nursing Practice* series is to bridge these gaps between the disciplines. The authors of the series are nurses or teachers of nurses and therefore have an intimate under-standing of nursing work and an appreciation of the importance of individualised nursing care. Yet at the same time, they are committed to a sociological outlook that asserts the salience of wider social forces to the work of nurses. The texts apply socio-logical theories and concepts to practical aspects of nursing. They explore nursing care as part of the social world, showing how different approaches to understanding the relationship between the individual and society have implications for nursing practice. By concentrating on a specific aspect of sociology or nursing, each book is able to provide the reader with a deeper knowledge of those aspects of sociology most pertinent to their own area of work or study. We hope that the series will encourage nurses to analyse critically their practice and profession, and to develop their own contribution to health care.

Margaret Miers, Sam Porter and Geoff Wilkinson

Acknowledgements

Intellectual projects of this size are rarely the result of an entirely individual effort, and this one is no exception. My colleagues, Ken Bishop, John Brewer, Denis O'Hearn, Sally Shortall and Jim Smyth, provided me with valuable insights and resources. My series editors, Margaret Miers and Geoff Wilkinson, gave me great support and encouragement. Margaret's speed of response to draft chapters, which were being produced under severe pressure of time, was much appreciated, as was the astuteness of her critical observations. Richenda Milton-Thompson at Macmillan must be congratulated for her great patience in the face of my continual procrastination. She showed considerable foresight in commissioning the series of books of which this is a part. I only hope that my efforts here justify her leap of faith.

At a more general level, I would like to thank all those researchers of nursing practice whose insights I recount. It was heartening indeed to see the quality of social theoretically informed work that is being done within the nursing arena.

Finally, I would like to mark my deep gratitude to Sandra Ryan. She not only acted as an unofficial editor, spending much precious time reading and commenting on each chapter as it fell from my personal computer, but also took up the domestic labour and child-caring slack that was an inevitable result of my attempt to write an entire book in 2 months. I do not deserve such generosity and good grace.

1 Introduction

Social theory has to be useful and useable; it is not an end in itself. The vexatious fact of society has to be tackled *in* theory *for* practice. These two tasks cannot be separated, for were practical utility to be the sole criterion we would commit ourselves to instrumentalism – to working with theoretically ungrounded rules of thumb. Conversely, a purely theoretical taming of the vexing beast may give a warm inner glow of ontological rectitude but is cold comfort to practical social analysts. They want a user-friendly tool kit and although it cannot come pocket-sized, customer services have every right to complain when handed an unwieldy device without any instructions on the assumption that if they handle it sufficiently this will somehow sensitize them to something.

(Archer 1995: 135)

Margaret Archer's statement well sums up the purpose of this book. Its aim is to move social theory into the daylight, so that it can be used with profit by nursing practitioners, students and researchers. In other words, I hope to show in as clear terms as possible how the 'vexing beast' of society impinges upon the practice of nursing and how an understanding of social theory will enable nurses to explore systematically the ways in which it impinges. However, such a bald statement begs a number of important questions. Before going any further, I feel I should answer five that strike me as particularly pertinent.

Question One: What is social theory?

Social theory consists of general approaches that seek to uncover and explain the nature and dynamics of social reality. The aim of social theory is not to describe specific instances in social life but to provide an overarching framework that can then be adopted to explain specific instances or general trends. These theories often concern themselves with ontology (questions concerning what the social world consists of), epistemology (questions concerning what we can know about the social world) and methodology (questions concerning the manner in which knowledge about the social world can be gained). As such, social theory provides the intellectual foundations for practical attempts to understand the world in which we live, in the form of sociological research. This answer may not strike you as entirely satisfactory; concise definition of social theory is far from easy. However, as you go through this book, I think that the sorts of issue that are addressed by social theory will become much clearer.

Question Two: Why 'social' theory rather than 'sociological' theory?

Once again, this is not any easy question to answer. My choice of 'social theory' lies in an uneasiness with the narrowness of the term 'sociological'. As you will see, throughout the book, my analysis leaks out from the narrow confines of the discipline of sociology to take account of issues that strictly belong in disciplines such as philosophy, political science, cultural theory and the history of ideas. It is to indicate the broadness of my approach that I use the term 'social theory'.

Question Three: What relevance do social theory and sociological research have to nursing practice?

The pertinence of sociology to nursing largely derives from the direction that nursing has taken in recent years. Not too long ago, it was thought that all that nurses needed to know were practical skills, along with some basic anatomy, physiology and pharmacology. This model of nursing knowledge was associated with an approach that is often described as the 'biomedical' model of health and illness, which saw health and illness as a purely mechanical, physical matter. However, in recent years, the biomedical model has been criticised for its narrow focus. In its place has emerged a model that spreads its explanatory net considerably wider. Instead of confining our interest in sick people to their internal pathologies, nurses now accept that persons' health status is determined by many factors, including their physical, cultural and social environment. Given the acceptance that social factors play a role in the determination of health and illness, there is a need for those involved in health care to understand the nature and effects of those factors, hence the need for sociological knowledge and, specifically, the social theories that ground that knowledge.

Question Four: Does social theory provide the kind of knowledge that nurses are able to use in order to inform their practice?

This question has come to the fore with the publication of an article by Keith Sharp (1994), who argued that sociology is an inappropriate form of knowledge for the practical activity of nursing. He asserts that because sociology is riven by disputes between competing theoretical positions, it is impossible to decide between their claims. As a result, practical health care actions cannot be based with any confidence upon sociological knowledge.

In relation to the observation that social theory is riven by disputes between theorists who adopt radically different interpretations of the social world, the first thing to note is that as you read through this book, you will quite quickly come to the realisation that this is indeed the case. However, does that mean they are unusable by nurses? My answer to this question has been 'no' on the grounds that nurses can use various criteria to decide which sociological approaches are most pertinent to their work (Porter 1995a). I identified three criteria, which, I argued, nurses can and do use when deciding what sort of knowledge (sociological or otherwise) is appropriate. The first criterion is termed 'pragmatic utility'. What is meant by this term is that nurses can judge the appropriateness of a sociological position according to its practical usefulness for the job of nursing. Quite simply, those ideas which nurses find most helpful in dealing with the practical day-to-day problems that they face are the ones that they are most likely to adopt. The second criterion I identified was 'philosophical compatibility' – the degree to which the philosophy underpinning a sociological perspective is compatible with nursing's own philosophy. The third and final criterion is that of 'ideological sympathy'. Here, I noted that nursing contained certain values and argued that these values can be used to judge which sociological perspectives are most sympathetic to nursing's concerns.

In summary, nurses are able to use their rational faculties to decide which variants of social theory are most pertinent to their practice. Moreover, there is no need for nurses to be dogmatic about this, choosing one theoretical position and rejecting all others. One of the things that I hope to show in this book is that there is something of use to be gained from all the social theories that I will consider and, indeed, many that I have not been able to include. That is not to say that I am without my own preferences and dislikes when it comes to social theories; I certainly am not. However, I have tried very hard (although probably not quite succeeded) to give each theory fair treatment.

Question Five: Is the approach currently adopted within nursing education towards social theory an adequate one?

The case against has been put forward by Hannah Cooke, who argues that sociology has been subverted by nursing educators. According to Cooke, the reasons for this subversion lie both in vested interests and matters of principle. At the level of interests, she posits that the ambitions of nursing's educational élite have led its members to blunt the critical edge offered by sociology (Cooke 1993a). At the level of principle, she argues that nursing's belief in the 'individualised care' of patients is incompatible with sociology, in that the unique message of the latter concerns the influence of social structure upon human behaviour (Cooke 1993b).

My response to this has been that there is a great deal of truth to this critique of nursing education. Indeed, one of the main purposes of this book is to contribute to efforts to rectify this problem. First of all, I hope it will demonstrate that self-criticism in the form of sociological reflection does not have to undermine nurses but can be used as a tool to understand nurses' social position in health care relationships. That knowledge then provides the potential both to improve care and to improve the social position of nurses in relation to that occupation which has traditionally enjoyed dominance in health care structures, namely medicine. Second, I hope to show, especially in Chapter 8, that it is possible to take due account of the importance of individual interactions while still addressing the issue of social structures.

The structure of the book

The book is divided into four parts, each of which has its own specific theme. Part I deals with the origins of social theory, looking at the ideas of the three dead men who are traditionally accredited as being the 'founding fathers' of sociology – Emile Durkheim, Karl Marx and Max Weber. What relevance, you may ask, have nineteenth-century sociological insights got for nurses finding themselves close to the twenty-first century? The answer to this question is that the positions that they outlined continue to this day to animate the various strands of social theory. While social theorists have attempted to update their ideas in order to tailor them to changing circumstances, their basic models about the nature of society continue to ground the approaches of many contemporary theorists.

Having established the 'baseline' of social theory in Part I, I go on to discuss a specific strand that has become increasingly influential in nursing knowledge, namely those positions which assert the need to look to individuals and their interactions if we are to understand the social world. This is the sort of approach of which Hannah Cooke was so suspicious. However, I hope to show that rather than simply being a vehicle for avoiding the social, these perspectives have much to offer us. I discuss three strands of what I will call action theories, namely symbolic interactionism, phenomenology and ethnomethodology – daunting names no doubt but hopefully considerably less daunting after you have read Part II.

At the opposite end of the theoretical spectrum to action theories is a position known as structuralism, which asserts the influence of social structures upon the thoughts and actions of individuals. The debate between structuralism and action theories is one that has dogged sociology for a long time. Another long-standing debate concerns the different interpretations of Western capitalism developed by Marx and Weber (which we will discuss in Part I). However, in recent years, attempts have been made to overcome such sterile divisions. These are the subject of Part III.

Chapter 7 focuses on attempts by critical theorists to adopt insights from both Marx and Weber, while Chapter 8 deals with two attempts to overcome the divide between social structure and social action, namely structuration theory and critical realism.

In contrast, there are those who have given up on trying to overcome the difficulties encountered by social theory as it has traditionally been constituted. They have argued that the dilemmas of social theory are insurmountable because of intrinsic flaws in the basic assumptions upon which social theory is founded. These approaches are the subject matter of Part IV, which deals both with feminism's critique of the male bias in sociology and postmodernism's attack on the rational assumptions that ground social theory.

The structure of chapters

I have written each chapter more or less according to a standard formula, although I have felt free to add variations to the theme whenever I feel it more appropriate. The formula involves starting the chapter with a general introduction to the social theory being addressed and then going on to discuss how that social theory has been, or might be, applied to health and health care issues. Finally, I take an example of nursing research that uses the theory in order to give a flavour of how it can shed light on our understanding of nursing practice. Each chapter concludes with a section that provides further readings for those who wish to delve deeper into that particular theory.

Sic men

Before starting with substantive issues, I would like to make a brief note on language. One of the problems that beset current sociological writers is the gendered nature of the English language. The traditional habit of using male pronouns to describe all human beings is now discredited. However, at least two problems remain. First, many of the writers quoted in the book wrote in an era when it was standard practice to use the male pronoun. What does one do with those quotations? One option is to place a (rather sanctimonious) 'sic' after every breach of non-sexist practice. It is not one I favour. The other problem relates to the alternatives to the male pronoun that have been developed. I have to say that I find devices such as 's/he' cumbersome and unappealing, not least because they are nigh on impossible actually to say. Thus, the option that I have chosen is to leave all the male pronouns in quotations as they are and to use exclusively female pronouns in my own writing.

PART I

Getting to the roots

One of the great difficulties of writing a history of ideas is deciding just where to start. It would be easy enough, for example, to go back to the Greeks, but I am not sure how much the socio-philosophical insights of Plato or Aristotle would be of use to twentieth-century nurses. More convincingly, I could have started at that point in history when the dynamics of social development became of intense intellectual interest, namely the eighteenth-century Enlightenment, or with the writings of the post-Enlightenment writer Auguste Comte (Andreski 1974), who is credited with inventing the term 'sociology'. However, while both Comte and the Enlightenment philosophers will be an integral part of our story, I have decided to view their ideas through the lens of those three great nineteenth- and early twentieth-century thinkers who are usually regarded as the founding fathers of modern sociology – Emile Durkheim, Karl Marx and Max Weber. The importance of these writers lies not just in what they had to say, although, as we shall see, they had much to say that remains pertinent to contemporary health care issues. Their importance also lies in the fact that the positions they staked out set the parameters for the evolution of social theory over the next century. This means that it is not possible to understand the ideas of contemporary theory without first of all having a grounding in the sociological classics.

One of the themes of this book is to trace the connections of ideas from the three founders down to the present day.

Durkheim's story is the briefest and will largely be confined to Chapter 2, which also includes discussion of the mid-twentieth-century American sociologist Talcott Parsons, who adopted and developed many of Durkheim's ideas.

Echoes of Marx, however, will rumble throughout the book, and we will hear them in the discussions on critical theory, critical realism and even feminism. Similarly, the ideas of Weber will be turn up again in our treatments of phenomenology and critical theory.

2 Structural functionalism and role theory

Introduction

Let me begin by briefly explaining the term 'structural functionalism' by taking each word in turn. 'Structuralist' sociological approaches are those which assert that the behaviour of people in society is structured according to a set of rules or laws. Evidence for this assertion is based on the observation that people do not act randomly; instead, their behaviour, including their social interactions, is patterned. Thus the aim of the sociologist is to identify the laws that structure our behaviour.

'Functionalism' in sociology is the view that society is a system made up of interconnected parts, each of which *functions* in a specific way to maintain that system as a whole. Perhaps the best way to illustrate functionalism is to use the metaphor of the body, society being regarded as working in a similar way to the human body. The body is made up of a number of organs, each of which plays a role in keeping the body alive. Thus, the renal system functions to assist fluid balance and to excrete unwanted chemicals, while the hypothalamus functions to ensure that the body maintains a constant temperature. Similarly, sociological functionalists argue that the family functions to train individuals into appropriate social roles, while health care professions function to ensure that the optimal health of members of society is maintained, so that they can go about their own functions within society to the best of their abilities.

Structuralism and functionalism were first combined by Emile Durkheim (1858–1917), who argued that sociologists should focus on two main aspects of the social system. First, they should attempt to uncover the social laws that structure the social world (this is the 'structural' bit). He saw social laws as being very similar to natural laws, such as gravity: just as gravity causes objects to fall to the ground, so social laws *cause* people to act in certain ways. However, Durkheim was interested in not only the causal relations involved in social laws, but also how the results of these causal relations impacted upon the social world. In other words, he saw the task of sociology as identifying the role played by the various social institutions such as the family, or the education system, which are the result of social laws, in maintaining the overall social system (the 'functionalism' bit):

> When, then, the explanation of a social phenomenon is undertaken, we must seek separately the efficient cause which produces it and the function it fulfils.
>
> (Durkheim 1938: 95)

Durkheim's ideas were further developed by the American sociologist Talcott Parsons (1902–79), whose work will be the subject of the latter half of this chapter. However, before launching into the murky depths of structural functionalism, it might be useful to set the scene by introducing Durkheim and Parsons, and indicating how I am going to use their ideas to address issues pertinent to nursing.

Emile Durkheim was the first person in France to be employed as a Professor of Sociology. His appointment at the Sorbonne in 1913 symbolised the fact that sociology had finally been given official recognition as a discipline in its own right. This was in no small part due to Durkheim's determination to demonstrate to the academic community that sociology was a rigorous scientific discipline. It is not possible to cover all the topics that Durkheim examined, which ranged from religion to politics and from methodology to mental health. Because of its pertinence to nursing and health care issues, my approach to his work will centre around his study of suicide. However, because his approach to suicide is deeply embedded in his more general social theory, it is necessary in the first instance to give a rather involved account of these theoretical foundations.

The influence of Talcott Parsons was almost as great as that of Durkheim. He held a position of unparalleled dominance in the discipline of sociology for approximately a quarter of a century between the 1940s and 1960s. During his career of over 50 years at Harvard, he developed what was regarded as the most systematic version of functionalist theory. While drawing heavily on the work of earlier European thinkers such as Durkheim and Weber, his influence decisively marked the dominant position that North America came to enjoy in the discipline of sociology during the mid-twentieth century. Parsons' output was enormous, and his writings were often highly complex and dense. Once again, it is not possible to give a comprehensive account of all aspects of his thought. As a result, I have opted to concentrate on his work on the medical and sick roles and how these might be interpreted in a nursing light. In order to examine how Parsons' construct of the medical role relates to the role of nurses, the nursing examples of Celia Davies' *Gender and the Professional Predicament in Nursing* (1995) and Titchen and Binnie's 'What am I meant to be doing? Putting practice into theory and back again in new nursing roles' (1992) are included. In relation to the notion of the sick role, Felicity Stockwell's *The Unpopular Patient* (1972) is addressed.

The Hobbesian problem of order

Before addressing these issues, it is necessary to set the scene by posing the question of how is it possible for individuals in society to come together to form a functioning whole, as sociological functionalists claim that they do. In other words, we must address the problem of social order, a question that was brought to the fore by a seventeenth-century English philosopher called Thomas Hobbes.

In his classic work *Leviathan* (1968 [1679]), Thomas Hobbes (1588–1679) began his interrogation of the problem of order by hypothesising what people would be like in a 'natural state', that is, a state in which social order had not been developed. He argued that in such a state, everyone would act according to their own individual passions and interests. This anarchic situation would automatically entail conflict between individuals: when different people desired the same object, they would become enemies. Being rational, they would adopt whatever means there were to hand to achieve their ends, and this would involve attempts to subjugate their rivals. Hobbes describes this rather unsavoury situation as follows: 'they are in that condition which is called Warre; and such a warre, as is of every man, against every man' (1968: 185). In his memorable phrase, this condition of war would lead to a life that is 'solitary, poore, nasty, brutish, and short' (1968: 186).

Hobbes argues that because humans are naturally rational and self-interested, it follows that a state of war of all against all is the natural state of humanity. In contrast, the social constraint of self-interest that is involved in the ordering of society is seen as an artificial construction. He asks how has it been possible for people to accept the imposition of a social order that constrains their rational pursuit of self-interest – how is the war of all against all avoided in normal social interaction? His answer is consistent with his assumption of individual rationality and self-interest. He argues that while immediate gratification may be gained by some in unconstrained competition, people realise the wider negative consequences of this in terms of its leading to a nasty, brutish and short existence. The 'natural state' of achieving self-interested goals is inefficient. A more effective route to gain safety and comfort is through order and the acceptance of authority. A state of peace is attained by people covenanting to each other that they will all accept the authority of a single ruling power – the 'Leviathan' – which will then have the capacity to impose peace and order.

Two things should be noted about Hobbes' answer to the question of social order. First, it was very individualistic: social order depends upon people seeing it in their own self-interest to co-operate with one another. Second, it conceived of order as being imposed by the state through coercion. Subsequent social analysts were less than happy with these assumptions.

Durkheim and social solidarity

Emile Durkheim rejected both of the above assumptions. He argued that a society is not simply an aggregation of self-interested individuals but rather consists of collective values, rules and norms that are external to individuals. This assertion of the existence of generalised social norms stands in contrast not only to Hobbes' individualism, but also to his conception of social order as being the product of state coercion.

It is worth taking some time to see how Durkheim came to this position. Following the earlier French sociologist Auguste

Comte (Andreski 1974), Durkheim adopted what is termed an emergent theory of reality. This view asserts that reality is constituted by a number of layers, each layer emerging from the interrelationship of the elements of a simpler level. However, an emergent level is not reducible to the simpler level from which it emerged. Take, for example, water, which is an emergent property resulting from the combination of two hydrogen atoms and one oxygen atom. The properties that water has, such as wetness, cannot be found in either hydrogen or oxygen on their own. The emergent theory of reality argues that from the physical emerges the chemical (in that chemical reactions emerge from activities of atomic particles), and on to the biological (life emerges from chemical reactions), the psychological (thought emerges from life) and, at the apex, the social (society emerges from the interaction of thinking individuals). The crucial point is that the properties of one level cannot be reduced to the properties of the one below. Thus, Durkheim argued that the social interaction of individuals leads to a 'collective consciousness' shared by most, if not all, members of society. This forms a social reality that has at least three unique properties, which in combination allow us to regard collective consciousness as a force that structures the social lives of individuals. First, collective consciousness pre-exists and outlives particular individuals. Second, it is felt by persons to be a general external force. Third, it is capable of shaping and constraining the actions of individuals (Durkheim 1938 [1901]).

A good example of what Durkheim is talking about is language. First, the English language existed long before any of us were born and is set to outlast us all. Second, the grammatical rules and lexicography of English are a general property used in the societies in which it is spoken, and their force upon members of society who are socialised into the use of English is unavoidable. Third, the nature of the English language constrains and shapes the way in which we can think and communicate. To take the well-known example of snow: English has relatively few words to describe snow and, as a result, English speakers' conceptualisations of that substance are fairly crude. In contrast, the Inuit language has a multiplicity of terms for it, which allows for a far more subtle and nuanced appreciation of something that is obviously very important in the lives of Inuits.

Collective consciousness and the division of labour

Probably the best way to illustrate how collective consciousness can affect the health of individuals is to use Durkheim's own work on suicide (Durkheim 1951 [1897]). Before doing so, however, it is necessary to ground the discussion in his more general analysis of the state of collective consciousness in industrialised societies, which is to be found in his book *The Division of Labour in Society* (1964 [1893]). As is apparent from the title he gave to the book, Durkheim saw the development of the division of labour that characterises modern societies as a key factor in explaining the characteristics of the collective consciousness.

In non-industrial societies, the tasks that people perform and the kind of lives they lead are often very similar. Thus, everyone would be responsible, either individually or collectively, for making their own clothes, growing their own food and rearing their own children. In contrast, industrialised societies are characterised by an increasing division of labour. Instead of people engaging in lots of tasks for fairly short periods of time, people tend to specialise in one task, for which they get paid. From the proceeds, they buy the products of other specialised workers' labours. We no longer make our own soap: we rely on people from Port Sunlight to do that. Indeed, it has come to the stage at which we very often do not even make our own dinner; instead, we rely on canteen workers or the manufacturers of ready-made meals.

Nor is it simply a matter of the division of labour: the communities and households in which we live have become less tightly knit. Durkheim wishes to explore what effect these socio-economic changes have had upon the nature of the collective consciousness. He argues that pre-industrialised societies are characterised by an all-embracing consensus, usually held together by a powerful religion. The way in which people behave is tightly controlled by shared values and beliefs. Society dominates the individual; people see themselves more as members of the collective than as individuals in their own right. In a rather poor analogy, Durkheim terms this form of collective consciousness 'mechanical solidarity', in that in such a situation, 'the social molecules [individuals]... could only operate in harmony in so far as they do not operate independently' (1964: 101). However, with the development of specialisation, a new form of solidarity develops, which depends not upon people's similarities, but upon their differences. This is termed 'organic solidarity', in that society becomes analogous with an organism, being constituted of differentiated organs, each with their own different and specific role to play. Here, collectively held values and beliefs become less important. In their place arises the morality of individualism, which asserts the importance of the individual. This is an important point often missed by critics of Durkheim. It was not that Durkheim denied the importance of individualism in favour of social structures but rather that he asserted that the very idea of the individual was the result of social development. In other words, organic solidarity does not mark the end of collective consciousness but merely the emergence of a new form of it.

As we shall see shortly, Durkheim regarded the rise of industrial society as creating tensions that did not exist under the collective consciousness of mechanical solidarity. These tensions were the result of *anomie* – the breakdown of social norms and moral obligations that has resulted from rapid social development. However, he saw the sort of industrialised society in which he lived as a period of transition. What was needed to reduce the tensions that Marx and others so graphically identified was the development of strong state regulation and the emergence of powerful occupational associations that would provide a buffer between the state and the individual.

Nevertheless, Durkheim recognised that the collective consciousness that currently existed created considerable problems. These problems were sufficiently severe to affect the emotional well-being of individuals. He explored this issue in *Suicide* (1951 [1897]). In this work, Durkheim examined a number of types of suicide, the one of most interest here being what he termed 'anomic suicide' – suicide that resulted from a lack of social integration.

Anomic suicide

Durkheim based his argument about anomic suicide on statistical information that he had gathered about suicide rates from a number of areas of Europe over a long period of time. From analysis of this data, he discovered two major trends. First, rates of suicide for particular populations tended to remain very stable from year to year. Second, there were significant differences in suicide rates between different countries and communities. This led him to conclude that killing oneself was not a purely individual matter: the likelihood of a person committing suicide was influenced by the society in which she lived. On further examination of the data, he uncovered a number of trends in the rates. These included evidence that suicide was more likely among city-dwellers than country-dwellers, unmarried men than married men, childless people than parents and Protestants than Catholics, who were in turn more likely to commit suicide than were Jews.

Durkheim's explanation for these trends rests on his argument that humans are by nature social animals. This means that they have a need to be part of a group; isolation leads to unhappiness, selfishness and anxiety. Thus, it is the anonymity of the city, as opposed to the tight-knit nature of rural communities, that leads more people living in urban areas to commit suicide. Similarly, if a man is unmarried, he is not integrated into a family unit. For Durkheim, the family functioned to strengthen social bonds and regulate sexual desire, thereby strengthening social solidarity and moral control. However, it should be noted that his statistics indicated that marriage was of benefit to *men's* mental health. For women, the story was different. While the overall statistics were not conclusive, Durkheim noted, in relation to the figures for France, that while married men were 1.5 times less likely to commit suicide than married men:

> in the same country the condition of a married woman was, on the contrary, made worse with respect to suicide unless the advent of children corrects the ill effects of marriage for her.

> (1951: 274)

This has led feminist commentators to argue that, while the family may be functional for men, in that it provides them with emotional support and domestic servicing, for women, who are expected to provide this support and servicing, getting married involves considerable restrictions and costs (Sydie 1987). More generally, this critique alerts us to the fact that we cannot automatically interpret social solidarity as being beneficial to all; we need also to consider on whose terms that solidarity has been constructed.

What about the religious pattern that Durkheim noticed? He makes a very similar argument, in that he observes that Protestantism is a highly individualistic religion. For Protestants, a person's relationship with God is direct and private, and participation in organised religion is not an essential component of their Christianity. In contrast, Roman Catholicism places a greater stress on collective worship and the institution of the Church. Here, a person's relationship with God is often mediated through officers of the Church, such as priests in confession. The Jewish religion stresses the importance of the community even more. For them, God's covenant is not with individual believers but with the Jewish people as a whole. Indeed, in most circumstances, it is obligatory that worship be conducted in a communal manner. Thus, Protestants are less socially integrated than Catholics, who are less integrated than Jews.

It is important to note that Durkheim is not claiming to be able to explain why particular individuals take their own life. What he is arguing is that, overall, there is an inverse relationship between the degree of integration in society and the rate of suicide in that society. The conclusion that might drawn from his work is that modern conditions of living are bad for mental health, and what is needed for improvement is a reincorporation of social solidarity into our collective consciousness – easier said than done! This is not a flippant point, for it leads to a gloomy assessment of the potential of health care interventions such as nursing having a significant impact upon the mental health of the population. As Taylor and Ashworth (1987) have pointed out, it is a mistake to interpret Durkheim as arguing that specific traits in society cause individual psychiatric problems. Rather, these problems emerge from the overall collective consciousness. This means that strategies geared towards mitigating or managing specific stressful factors are unlikely to be very successful. However, on a more optimistic note, Taylor and Ashworth argue that Durkheim is not asserting that the modern collective consciousness is an unmitigated disaster for our health – it has both costs and benefits:

> the increasing individualism and autonomy, which is part of the process generating the stressful conditions of modern life, also liberated individuals from the yolk of tradition, and brought about those improvements that McKeown (1976) and others have linked with the modern rise of population.

> (1987: 50)

Durkheim's positivism

Before moving on, I should point out that not everyone has been convinced by the methodology of Durkheim's research of anomic suicide. It is argued that this was tainted by the assumptions of positivism. Positivism is a theory of knowledge developed by Auguste Comte (Andreski 1974), who saw sociology as being the science of society, just as physics is a science of the natural world, the aim of both being to identify the mechanical relations of cause and effect that cause events to occur. Comte rejected the validity of religious explanations of first causes and ultimate ends, arguing that they relied on unverifiable speculation. For him, knowledge did not come from faith or revelation but through the systematic identification of facts using scientific method. Thus, the only valid form of knowledge is knowledge of things about which we can be 'positive'. Positivism as a philosophy of science is closely linked to what is termed 'empiricism' – the belief that all knowledge comes from experience. However, it differs from empiricism in that it posits that all knowledge comes from a combination of theory and experience, theory being essential to the process of making sense of the ordering of the world. Specifically, positivism accepts the possibility of identifying general laws that govern the events that we experience. For Comte, social laws were as invariable as natural laws. He therefore placed a great deal of emphasis on social order, arguing that people should resign themselves to obeying social laws, just as they are resigned to natural laws such as the force of gravity.

By way of a slight diversion, it might be noted that Florence Nightingale was heavily influenced by the ideas of Comte. While rejecting Comte's dismissal of Christianity, she accepted his conception of the invariance of both natural and social laws:

> His moral and His physical law stand on exactly the same basis: neither is ever broken: bodies do not fall upwards; and His moral law which says 'if you kill, certain consequences will follow, and if certain circumstances take place you will kill', is always kept.
>
> (Nightingale 1860: 303–4)

According to Nightingale, these laws determined the require-ments of health, and if these requirements were not met, disease resulted. It was on this basis that she argued that the role of nurses was to 'put the patient in the best condition for nature to act upon him' (1970 [1859]: 75). For her, the laws of nursing were one and the same as moral and natural laws (van der Peet 1995).

Since Nightingale's time, positivism has continued to exert considerable influence over nursing's approach to research. However, as we shall see in later chapters, positivism's position in nursing research has been challenged in recent years by more inter-pretative approaches to the problems of health.

The interpretative critique of suicide

Interpretative sociologists such as Atkinson (1971) are sceptical about Durkheim's attempt to analyse suicide through positivist scientific methods. Specifically, they question his acceptance of statistical information. Atkinson argues that Durkheim does not take account of the beliefs, meanings and motives of the people involved in constructing these statistics. Durkheim gets his 'facts' from adding up coroners' decisions about the cause of death. While he does not assume that these will always be correct, he does assume that by using large numbers of decisions, mistakes will cancel each other out. However, in uncertain cases (of which there are very many), coroners have to use subjective evaluation to make a decision. They usually do this by attempting to discover the state of mind of the deceased prior to her death. In order to do this, they ask family and friends. With all the guilt and shame that is experienced by bereaved family members, it is likely that they will tend to play down the interpretation of the death as suicide. In contrast, single people are less likely to have others close to them with a vested interest in interpreting their death as an accident. Similarly, in close rural communities, the suicide is more likely to be known by the coroner, who will therefore have a personal motivation for not attaching the stigma of suicide. In terms of religion, it might be argued that different religions stigmatise suicide to greater or lesser degrees. In a religious community where suicide is highly stigma-tised, there will be greater pressure on coroners to place a more benign interpretation on deaths that were possibly due to suicide – who wants to be responsible for condemning someone to eternal fire and brimstone?

Leabharlann
Contae na Midhe
5155 321

The pertinence of Durkheim to nursing

Durkheim's work allows us to step back and put into perspective nursing's position in the overall nature of things. His idea of the collective consciousness suggests that health and illness are not simply matters of individual responsibility. The types of illness we suffer from and the amount of sickness that occurs is to a large extent a social product. It follows from this that while health care workers such as nurses can help or ameliorate the suffering of specific individuals, their capacity to make general changes to the health of populations is constrained by the nature of the society in which they work. For example, the balance of stress and well-being that exists in modern Western societies is to a considerable extent fixed by the social organisation of those societies through its influence upon the consciousness of societies' members. Consideration of Durkheim encourages modesty, in that acceptance of his arguments might lead us to conclude that while nursing has the capacity to help specific individuals with the problems that the world throws upon them, it does not have the capacity on its own to change the world.

Parsons' structural functionalism

Parsons was much influenced by the work of Durkheim in his examination of the problem of social order. His grounds for disagreeing with Hobbes were very similar. He argued that social order could not depend on something as precarious as naked self-interest. For social order to succeed, members of society needed to share a moral commitment to the rules of society. The basis for social co-operation lay in a consensus of values between members. He saw Durkheim's achievement as having identified the structure of society as being 'formed mainly by a common system of normative rules which... rest upon a system of ultimate common value attitudes' (Parsons 1937: 464). Thus, the values that people hold to are not purely a matter of individual conscience. This denial of the individuality of values is at odds with common sense: most of us believe that we are, as individuals, responsible for the values that we hold. One of Parsons' main aims was to defend such a counterintuitive concept of values. His answer lay in the process of *socialisation*, the process whereby individuals learn to accept the common values of society on what goals, and what actions to attain those goals, are appropriate. Socialisation starts at birth, when children begin to learn the expectations that others will have of them. The primary social institutions involved in socialisation are the family and the education system. Because we are exposed to socialisation from the very start of our lives, we take for granted the values that we learn; in Parsons' terms, they become *internalised*. It is in this way that our commitments as individuals become integrated with the wider norms and values in society.

Parsons (1951) argued that social expectations are translated into action through the learning of social roles. Thus, through the influence of socialising institutions, we learn how to play various roles that we will be required to adopt during our lives. A role is a combination of normative expectations relating to the rights and duties of an individual in a given social position. In other words, it involves expectations of how we should interact with others. When particular roles are generally accepted by large numbers of people, they become *institutionalised*. For Parsons, social institutions are essentially clusters of social roles that share common foundational values. Societies in which roles are highly institutionalised enjoy a great deal of consensus among their members. Conversely, where roles are not generally accepted, society is characterised by anomie.

The benefits of the institutionalisation of roles, according to Parsons, is that they lead to a stable social system, characterised by an equilibrium between the various parts of society. For a society to survive, the institutions of which it is composed have to function in a way that will promote its survival. The functional needs of societies are twofold: there must be internal cohesion within the system and there must be a successful relationship between the system and its external environment. Thus, for example, the institution of the family has an integrative function in society, promoting social cohesion, while economic institutions function to convert natural resources into goods.

So far, the ideas of Parsons that we have been discussing have been very general in their nature. However, Parsons sought to go beyond these general typologies of the nature of society and be more explicit about the roles and institutions that he argued were so essential to the functioning of society. He argued that it was possible to classify the values that provided the foundation for these roles and institutions. While the number of particular values that may be embedded in a role is almost infinite, Parsons held that these values could all be categorised within a limited number of general 'pattern variables'. He argued that values underlying any action within a role could be seen as either *instrumental* or *expressive*. Instrumental actions are those which are goal oriented; in other words, they are actions that are means to an identified end. Conversely, expressive actions are those which are performed for their own sake: they are an end in themselves. On the basis of this dichotomy, Parsons posited five alternative sets of pattern variable, which, he argued, structured all social actions:

EXPRESSIVE	INSTRUMENTAL
Affectivity	Affective neutrality
Collective orientation	Self-orientation
Particularism	Universalism
Ascription	Achievement
Diffuseness	Specificity

The first dichotomy of pattern variables is between affectivity and affective neutrality. This refers to the degree to which emotional involvement animates a role. If a role is affective, the person's relations with others are highly emotional, whereas if it is affectively neutral, interaction is unemotional and impersonal. The role of a mother in relation to her child might be an example of affectivity, whereas the role of a traffic warden in relation to motorists might be seen as affectively neutral.

The second dichotomy is between collective orientation versus self-orientation. This relates to whether people put the interests of the group to which they belong before their own interests (collective orientation) or whether they primarily pursue their own individual interests (self-orientation). Kamikaze pilots might be regarded as having a high degree of collective orientation, while loan sharks might be seen as more self-orientated.

The third dichotomy, particularism versus universalism, refers to how people respond to others. In particularism, individuals act differently towards different people, depending on how much they feel they have in common. It involves the subjective evaluation of others. In universalism, people act towards others according to general principles, irrespective of how they view them as individuals. This entails objective valuation. If one is asking for a loan from one's bank manager, the manager's response in deciding whether to grant the loan on the basis of a formal assessment of one's credit-worthiness would be an example of universalism, in that everyone she deals with would be assessed on the same grounds. Alternatively, if one asked for a loan from one's sister, she might be expected to take a more particularistic approach that was influenced by her sense of family loyalty (or, on the other hand, she might not!).

The fourth pattern variable, ascription versus achievement, relates to the manner in which status is accorded to people. With ascription, people are ascribed a status according to what are seen as intrinsic qualities (or a lack of them), whereas with achievement, their status relates to their performance in achieving certain goals. For example, members of the British royal family are ascribed positions of wealth and privilege simply because of whom they were born to, irrespective of how good they are at being royal. Conversely, professional footballers achieve their star status through prowess on the playing pitch.

The final variable is diffuseness versus specificity. In a diffuse role, the relationship that a person has within that role will cover a wide range of interests. In a specific role, the relationship is restricted to particular areas. Parenthood might be regarded as a diffuse role in that it involves feeding, clothing, nurturing, teaching and so on, while working on a supermarket checkout entails a high degree of role specificity in that one's relationship with customers is limited to the business of calculating the price of the goods they wish to purchase and then extracting that price.

It should be noted that Parsons did not regard these opposing sets of variables in a neutral fashion. He saw instrumental variables as being associated with 'advanced' societies, public life and men, while expressive variables were associated with 'primitive' societies, private life and women. It is strongly implicit in Parsons' analysis that the former set of pattern variables is superior to the latter. An illustration of this can be seen in his use of doctors as an example to demonstrate how mid-twentieth-century North American male professional roles were functional for that society.

The pattern variables of the medical role

According to Parsons (1951), doctors, if they are playing their role appropriately, embody four of the five instrumental pattern variables. They are affectively neutral, in that it is inappropriate for them to have emotional, sentimental or sexual ties to their patients. They are universal in their approach, adopting an objective, scientific stance that involves choosing the most effective means to treat their patients. These means are chosen irrespective of the personal characteristics of the person whom they are treating. Their role is highly orientated towards achievement, in that it is through demonstrating their knowledge and technical skills after long years of training that doctors gain their right to practise. Finally, they adhere to role specificity, in that they are orientated solely to the health of their patients and do not interfere in other areas of their lives, which are the responsibility of other experts.

The exception to the instrumental rules of doctoring is that of collective orientation. This is what marks doctors out from those professionals involved in private business. Because of their professional responsibilities, doctors are required to perform the public service of promoting health rather than be orientated towards the pursuit of profit. The obvious response to this portrayal of doctors as altruistic agents, unconcerned about self-advancement, is, if this is the case, how come they have managed to succeed in gaining so much status and remuneration? The functionalist reply to this question is that they have gained their rewards because of their important functional position within society. Barber argues that, because the knowledge and skills of professions such as medicine are so important to the well-being of society:

> orientation primarily to community interest rather than individual interest is an essential attribute of professional behavior. Individual self-interest is, of course, not utterly neglected in professional behavior, but is subserved *indirectly*.
>
> (1963: 672)

According to Barber, the problem of conflict between self- and community interest is solved by society rewarding professionals with money and, more importantly, status in return for adopting a collective orientation in their work. This rationalisation of professional status on the grounds of the functional benefits that professions provide for society as a whole has not convinced everyone. Rueschemeyer (1964) argues that such a position is based on at least two highly questionable assumptions: first, that all members of 'society' will benefit equally from the knowledge and skills of professionals; and second, that all members of society will share equally the central values of professionals. He also notes that the process by which professionals are imbued with an altruistic collective orientation in return for society's gifts is entirely mysterious.

Nursing example: gender and professional roles

Parsons' use of pattern variables to locate professions such as medicine can also be subjected to feminist analysis. While she does not directly address Parsons and his pattern variables, Celia Davies, in her book *Gender and the Professional Predicament in Nursing* (1995), puts forward a critique of the medical model of professionalism, thereby challenging his assumptions about the benefits of instrumental role formations. Davies argues that what she calls 'cultural codes of gender' structure the way in which people see the world and act within it. She uses the term 'cultural code' to distinguish her position from *biological determinism*, which asserts that the differences in the way in which men and women think and act can be explained by their biological make-up, and from *social determinism*, which sees gender roles as being determined by socialisation. In contrast, cultural codes provide the context within which people develop, but they do not necessarily map on to specific individuals in a straightforward manner; women can be influenced by the male cultural code and vice versa. Davies argues that the cultural code of masculinity is dominant in the public world. This code places value on self-esteem, autonomy, control over the world and mastery of others. In contrast, the subordinate feminine cultural code places value on selflessness, relatedness, understanding and group orientation. Ironically, while masculinity proclaims itself as superior, men could not go about their activities in the public world if their personal and domestic needs were not fulfilled by women.

Davies identifies the medical profession as a product of the masculine cultural code. Each of the instrumental pattern variables so valued by Parsons can be seen as reflecting a masculine view of the world:

> Achievement: 'Professional knowledge is gained by dint of a lengthy and heroic individual effort. The effort is a project involving mastery, resulting in knowledge as a "possession" of the autonomous individual.'
>
> (1995: 59)

> Specificity: 'The profession shapes and controls knowledge... It creates specializations, celebrating depth rather than breadth. Specialists, with their command and again mastery of an area, are more highly regarded than generalists.'
>
> (1995: 59)

> Universalism: 'What is apparently attention to the fullest circumstances of the client/case, is in practice a sifting of information in terms of a diagnostic model and a translation into categories of action that fit the competencies of the professional. Universal values are assumed.'
>
> (1995: 59)

> Affective neutrality: 'The portrayal of a professional concern... keeps emotion at a distance – the lack of emotional display in the delivery of skill is a valued aspect of professionalism. Professionals offer a detached "understanding" when clients, in what can be a highly charged context, frequently apologise for their fears and their tears.'
>
> (1995: 59–60)

It can be seen that the converse of Parsons' construction of the medical role is that nursing is expected to be the feminine adjunct to this masculine professional project. By taking on the feminine 'duties' of caring and domestic labour, nursing allows medicine 'to present itself as masculine/rational and to gain the power and privilege of so doing' (Davies 1995: 61). Given the gendered nature of professionalism, Davies concludes that:

Nursing's long-term project may therefore be not to become a profession in the present sense of this term, but to challenge the gendered basis of this concept.

(1995: 61)

Interestingly, Davies does not go down the path followed by a number of feminist commentators (such as Gilligan, 1982, whom we will meet in Chapter 9) on differences between masculinity and femininity, which is to invert the current valuation of these cultural codes by presenting the feminine in a positive light. Instead, she seeks to go beyond gendered thinking and the limitations it entails for both sexes. She proposes a new nursing practitioner who is:

- neither distant nor involved but *engaged*;
- neither autonomous nor passive/dependent but *interdependent*;
- neither self-oriented nor self-effacing but accepting of an *embodied use of self* as part of the therapeutic encounter;
- neither instrumental nor passive but a *creator of an active community* in which a solution can be negotiated;
- neither the master/possessor of knowledge nor the user of experience but a *reflective user of experience and expertise*.

(Davies 1995: 149–50)

New nursing roles

These proposals for values to underlie the nursing role are consonant with many of the ideas being put forward by proponents of 'new nursing' (Salvage 1990). They involve a tempering of the previously dominant instrumental approach to nursing work through the inclusion of more open, expressive modes of activity. Such a change in the nursing role is far from easy to realise, as is illustrated by Titchen and Binnie's (1992) case study of the move to patient-centred practice. The development of closer and more sustained relationships between nurses and patients was promoted through a restructuring of nursing roles.

This was primarily effected through two structural changes to the organisation of nursing work, namely the introduction of team nursing, whereby patients were allocated to a specific team of nurses for their stay in hospital, and primary nursing, whereby each patient was provided with an individual nurse to take overall responsibility for their care. Both these developments entailed a flattening of the hierarchical structure of the ward, which involved a devolution of power and responsibility from ward managers to staff nurses. The introduction of these new roles was not without its problems, the most serious of which was the development of *role ambiguity*, which meant that neither senior nor junior staff were clear about what their rights and obligations were in the new order of things. Old ways of thinking about hierarchical roles were hard to shed. Thus, the new team co-ordinators on the one hand were unsure of their authority in relation to the ward sister, but on the other adopted a traditional hierarchical role in relation to the other members of their team. As a result of their findings, Titchen and Binnie argue that because the tendency is to revert to old certainties, it is not enough to allow new roles to evolve in an unco-ordinated fashion:

> Clinical leaders need to be very explicit about the strategies they are adopting. It cannot be assumed that people will be able to clarify roles, accept responsibilities and fulfil new obligations without the development of new skills. The evidence suggests that staff development early in an innovation is necessary. New roles, their responsibilities, obligations and boundaries need to be clarified and skilfully negotiated and facilitated.
>
> (1992: 1060)

Consideration of Titchen and Binnie's work might lead us to conclude that while Parson's description of the pattern variables underlying professional work might be less than appropriate for nursing, his more general point about the fundamental importance of social roles that involve normative expectations relating to the rights and duties of an individual in a given social position continues to have pertinence for the understanding of evolving nursing roles.

The sick role

In line with his belief that central to social roles were relationships with others, Parsons, in addition to examining the role of the doctor, also addressed the role of the patient in his famous conceptualisation of the sick role. Given the social context in which it was developed, Parsons' (1951) notion of the sick role was a radical one. At the time when he was writing, the dominant interpretation of illness was based on the medical model, with its assumption that being sick was a purely biological matter. In contrast to this taken-for-granted interpretation, Parsons argued that sickness was a profoundly social phenomenon, in that illness behaviour was the product of the general values of a society. In Western societies, which place so much emphasis on activity, individual responsibility and achievement, to be sick is seen as not being able to work (Turner 1987). On this basis, Parsons argued that if social rules about sickness behaviour were too lax, this would put considerable strain upon the productive capacities of society. In other words, strict norms about the sick role were essential in order to prevent sickness from becoming dysfunctional for the achievement of social goals (Mechanic 1968).

Parsons argued that there were four aspects to the sick role in Western societies. First, it involved legitimate withdrawal from the normal requirements of social life such as work. Second, those taking on the sick role were not seen as responsible for their condition. However, to balance these rights, there were also obligations, the first being the obligation to do all in one's power to get better, from which led the final aspect – the obligation to seek and accept health care from a competent health care practitioner.

A number of criticisms have been levelled at Parsons' conception of the sick role. It has been pointed out that the model is only really pertinent to unproblematic acute illnesses, in that it assumes that people will get better (Turner 1987). In chronic illnesses, people may be either permanently removed from the workforce as a result of incapacity (for example after a cerebrovascular accident) or forced to accept commitments despite the fact that they are ill (for example those suffering from diabetes mellitus).

Another criticism revolves around Parsons' assumption of the unproblematic (albeit unequal) relationship between medical practitioners and their patients. This rests upon his assumption that social norms, if they are properly institutionalised, tend to be universally held by all members of a society. Thus, the fourth aspect of the sick role is that the person adopting the role accepts the medical interpretation of what is wrong and what should be done about it. This portrayal of consensus between patient and physician has been challenged by Freidson (1970), who argues that because they view illness from differing perspectives, the relationship between doctors and patients is very often one of conflict rather than consensus. One of the ways in which this conflict manifests itself is through health care workers typifying patients as 'bad patients' (Murcott 1981).

Nursing example: the unpopular patient

The potential for conflict between health care workers and their patients was highlighted by Felicity Stockwell in *The Unpopular Patient* (1972). While Stockwell's treatment of Parsons' idea of the sick role is only tangential to her work, it is possible to take a more explicitly Parsonian interpretation of her findings. Stockwell found that the patients in her study whom nurses least enjoyed looking after were those who did not conform to the role expectations that the nurses felt appropriate for a hospitalised patient. Specifically, unpopular patients were usually those who the nurses felt exaggerated their needs and whose condition was not seen as being severe enough to warrant admission. Neither the 'moaners'' nor the 'hypochondriacs'' claims to be accepted into the sick role were seen as valid by the nurses studied. They were not regarded as discharging their responsibility to co-operate with health care workers to get well as soon as possible. In response to this, nurses adopted a number of sanctions that entailed reducing the privileges that are attendant upon adoption of the sick role. Thus, they ignored patients, 'forgot' their requests, refused to do favours, rigidly enforced rules and interacted with these patients in a sarcastic manner.

Assessing Parsons' role theory

Consideration of *The Unpopular Patient* suggests that, once again, it might be wise for nurses to accept Parsons' insights in a qualified way. It is certainly the case that people adopt roles in life such as the nursing role and the patient role, and that those roles carry with them social expectations about appropriate behaviour. Uncovering and understanding the nature of those roles is certainly a useful exercise. However, part of that understanding should be of whose expectations are involved. Parsons' analysis seems to work on the assumption of consensus – that there is general agreement about roles. However, we cannot assume that what is functional for one group will be functional for another. In this case, nurses' expectations of the role that patients should play, and their responses to those who did not adopt that role, indicates that such a construction of the sick role posed serious problems for some patients. While it is possible for structural functionalism to account for conflict (Merton 1968), the use of Parsons' role theory in relation to health care does not allow us fully to interrogate issues of power and inequality between professionals and clients. As we shall see in the next chapter, other perspectives take considerably more account of the importance of inequality and conflict in society.

Recommended further reading

A brief account of Emile Durkheim's work has been written by Anthony Giddens (1978), who has also edited a useful book on positivism (Giddens 1974). A more in-depth treatment of Durkheim is provided by Steven Lukes (1973), while Taylor and Ashworth (1987) apply his theories to the sociology of health. A brief description of Parsons' sociology is given by Hamilton (1983). A discussion of the criticisms of functionalism is given by Cohen (1968), while a defence of his concept of the sick role can be found in Gerhardt (1987).

3 Marxism and the political economy of health

Introduction

The focus of this chapter is on the ideas of Karl Marx (1818–83) and how they have influenced our understanding of health and health care. As the chapter's title indicates, Marxist approaches to health care emphasise that they cannot be divorced from wider political considerations, which are in turn deeply influenced by economic arrangements.

After a broad review of the ideas of Karl Marx, this chapter will proceed to examine how his ideas have been applied to issues concerning health, illness and health care. This will be done under three broad headings. The first approach involves a critique of the economic inequalities generated by capitalism, and a linkage between those inequalities and inequalities in health. The second approach examines how the provision of health care tends to function for the benefit of capitalism. The final approach involves a criticism of health care industries on the grounds that their prime purpose is to make profits out of people's illnesses, which means that they will often not develop the most effective forms of care because they are not as lucrative as other, less effective interventions. A nursing example of how Marxist thought can be used to interrogate practice is found in Bridges and Lynam's 'Informal carers: a Marxist analysis of social, political, and economic forces underpinning the role' (1993).

Karl Marx

It is difficult to categorise Marx into a single academic discipline; as well as being a social theorist, he was a philosopher, economist, political scientist and revolutionary activist. Born in Germany of Jewish stock, his political activities led to persecution and a move to Paris. He was subsequently expelled from France and settled in

London, where much of his intellectual work was carried out in the hallowed surroundings of the British Museum reading room. A good deal of his work was carried out in collaboration with his friend and benefactor, Friedrich Engels (1820–95).

When people think of Karl Marx, they often think of communism and the communist regimes of eastern Europe and Asia, which have now either rejected or modified out of all recognition what they used to claim was the practical implementation of his philosophy. However, the influence of Marx stretches far beyond practical politics: it has also made an enormous contribution to the way in which people think about the social world. As Peter Singer noted:

> Can anyone now think about society without reference to Marx's insights into the links between economic and intellectual life? Marx's ideas brought about modern sociology, transformed the study of history, and profoundly affected philosophy, literature and the arts. In this sense of the term – admittedly a very loose sense – we are all Marxists now.
>
> (1980: 1)

The purpose of this chapter is to explore whether Marxist ideas have anything useful to say in relation to nursing and health care. This will be done first of all by examining the ideas of Marx himself, then considering how Marxists have applied his ideas to issues concerning health and finally looking at how they might usefully be used in explaining aspects of nursing practice.

Historical materialism

Central to Marx's work is the attempt to understand how the human world develops and changes over time. Marx saw human society as an evolving process. He argued that, in order to understand the world, it was necessary to understand those forces which drive this process of transformation. For Marx, these forces are not external to the world we live in – it is not 'God' or 'destiny' that leads the social world to develop in the way it does. Instead, change is generated by internal tensions, or 'contradictions', within societies. Therefore, in order to understand the world, it is not enough simply to look at surface events. The social scientist needs to look deeper than external appearances in order to uncover the underlying tensions that provide the potential for change. By arguing in this way, Marx is not rejecting the traditional scientific activity of searching out 'facts'. What he is arguing is that this is only the first stage of the process of scientific analysis. In the philosophical jargon of the day, Marx argued that science should take a 'dialectical' approach. A dialectical process involves a contradiction between two forces and the resolution that develops as a result of their clash. This is rather different from the traditional scientific understanding of how change takes place. In traditional science, change is seen as a matter of cause and effect, one force making another event happen. In contrast to cause and effect, dialectics involves interaction – both contradictory forces affect each other, producing an effect that is qualitatively different from either of them. This is significant because it entails a rejection of determinism – the philosophy that all events, including human actions, are determined by outside forces (in other words, that they are just the effects of prior causes). For dialecticians, such a position oversimplifies the complex interactions that are involved in human societies made up of thinking individuals. However, a dialectical position also involves a rejection of pure chance or complete free will, in that it sees the direction of events in society as being shaped by underlying tensions or contradictions.

Marx got the idea of the dialectics of change from the German philosopher W.G.F. Hegel. However, in his own famous phrase, he turned Hegel 'on his head'. Hegel saw dialectical development in terms of ideas. Marx did not accept that ideas were fundamental. He rejected the philosophical position of 'idealism', which assumes that the phenomena of the human mind constitute the ultimate reality. Instead, he was a materialist. In broad terms, materialism contends that whatever exists is, or depends upon, matter – that the physical world is the ultimate reality. Marx's materialism was of a special kind. He believed that what made humans unique – what made them stand out from animals – was their capacity to mould the physical world to their own ends. In other words, humans are able to take the raw materials of the physical world and work on them to make them into things of use: houses, heating systems, beds, soluble insulin, the list is endless. This insight led Marx to stress the central importance of labour, arguing that the human activities of production and reproduction is what gives us our uniqueness or 'species being'. This labour does not take place any old how: it is organised in very specific ways – work is organised by certain social relationships. Thus, Marx's materialism included both the physical world (both in its raw and worked-upon state) and the social relations in which people are organised in production. In order to understand change and development, he argued that it was necessary to uncover the tensions and contradictions within this material world that were the dynamos for change; to understand history is to identify the dialectics of production (Marx 1946 [1889]).

Marx distinguished two aspects of production: the forces of production and the relations of production. There are three aspects to the forces of production:

1. the physical objects that make up the raw materials of production;
2. labour power: the human activity that works upon those raw materials to make them into things of use;
3. the means of production: the machinery and technology that people use when labouring.

The relations of production concern peoples' social position in relation to production. For Marx, the fundamental division in society was between those who owned and controlled the means of production and those who did not. It was along this fault line that he divided society into two classes.

One cannot overemphasise the importance that Marx places on economic relations. It is upon their base that the entire edifice of society is constructed: political structures, laws, even the way in which people think, are all grounded in the relations of production:

In the social production of their life, men enter into definite relations that are indispensable and independent of their will, relations of production which correspond to a definite stage of development of their material productive forces. The sum total of these relations of production constitutes the economic structure of society, the real foundation, on which rises a legal and political superstructure and to which correspond definite forms of social consciousness. The mode of production of material life conditions the social, political and intellectual life process in general. It is not the consciousness of men that determines their being, but, on the contrary, their social being that determines their consciousness.

(Marx 1970: 80)

The forces of production are always developing – new technologies and ways of working are always being introduced. Marx argues that this leads to tensions between the new forces of production and the relations of production that developed under the old forces of production. For example, the feudal system of a small aristocracy, who owned and controlled the means of production, and a large serfdom developed during an era when poor communications systems meant that the only viable form of economy was a local one. However, with improved transport (and therefore trading) and the rise of factories and cities, the old system in which people were tied to their lord and master became outdated. The new forces of production required a more mobile and flexible workforce. This led to a tension between the new, industrial and mercantile forces of production and the old feudal relations of production. Out of this tension emerged a new social relationship – capitalism. What is unique about capitalism is that involves 'free' labour. In feudalism, the lord literally owned the labourer. In capitalism, the factory owners (the bourgeoisie or capitalists) only own the factories and not the people who work in them. Instead, the workers (or proletariat) are formally free to decide to whom they are going to sell their labour. However, because they have no choice but to sell their labour to someone, this is not true freedom but a new form of oppression, which Marx called wage slavery. Nevertheless, because capitalism freed up the relationship between individual workers and capitalists, it was a far more flexible and competitive relation of production, better able to cope with and encourage technological and productive advances.

It is often assumed that Marx was totally critical of capitalism, but that is not quite the case (Sowell 1986). Marx recognised that, with capitalism, there was, for the first time in history, the technological capacity to enable all the people of the earth to live in material comfort. However, he also recognised that within capitalism, this potential was not, and would not be, realised. Marx identified at least four crucial faults with capitalism:

1. Exploitation

This involves the question of where the wealth of the owners of the means of production comes from. Marx's answer was that it is created by the labour of the proletariat. By turning raw materials into manufactured products, workers are adding value to those raw materials. Yet, they do not get the full benefits of that value addition. They sell their labour at a certain price to capitalists, who will pay the lowest wages that the market can bear. There is therefore no connection between the value that the workers create through their labour and the wages that they earn. Capitalists pocket the difference. It is through this 'surplus value' that capital is accumulated. Therefore, Marx argued, capital is nothing more than accumulated labour. In other words, capitalists get rich by exploiting workers.

2. Alienation

We have already seen how Marx believed that what makes us human is the capacity to shape the world in which we live – that it is in the activities of producing their world that humans' 'species being' lies. However, under capitalism, workers lose control of their work. Someone else tells them what to make and how to make it, and when they have made it, it does not belong to them. This means that workers are estranged or alienated from their own labour. For Marx, this has profound consequences. Because it is our capacity to work on our environment to change it to our own ends (our capacity to labour) that makes us human, if we are alienated from our labour, we are also alienated from our humanity. Thus, for Marx, capitalism is not simply bad because it involves the exploitation of workers. Far more profound, he argues, is the fact that capitalism prevents us from developing as human beings. It produces alienation (Marx 1959 [1844]).

3. Private property

At the root of the evils of exploitation and alienation lies the ownership of private productive property. As we have noted, Marx argued that the class division between the ownership and non-ownership of the means of production is the fundamental division in society. This division provides the dialectical tension that drives history forward. As long as it remains, there will be social conflict. This is because the owners are obliged to exploit the non-owners in order to maintain their property, while the non-owners are driven to challenge ownership because it involves their own exploitation and alienation. It was for these reasons that Marx stated at the start of the *Communist Manifesto* that 'The history of all hitherto existing society has been the history of class struggle' (Marx and Engels 1967 [1888]: 79).

4. Forces of production

According to Marx, capitalism's very success was going to be its downfall. As capitalism grows and expands, industry becomes concentrated in huge enterprises, which can no longer be controlled by individual capitalists. Increasingly large numbers of people are required to run modern businesses. In Marxist jargon, the forces of production become increasingly socialised. Yet capitalism involves the private ownership of property. There is therefore an increasing contradiction between the socialised nature of the forces of production and the private nature of the means of production. This contradiction provides the motor for socialism which involves socialised ownership and control.

The promise of communism

For Marx, the end of exploitation and alienation will only be achieved with the end of the private productive property. With the advent of capitalism, the forces of production to enable such a development are created. Thus, the end to the dialectical cycles of class struggle will involve the overthrow of the propertied bourgeoisie by the propertyless proletariat. Thus, the promise of communism is the end of exploitation, alienation and class conflict through the abolition of private ownership of the means of production.

Marxist explanations of ill health

Marx's writings on the specific issue of health are rather scattered – he made no systematic examination of the issue. However, the Marxist approach to health and illness is well summed up by his close collaborator, Friedrich Engels:

When one individual inflicts bodily injury upon another, such injury that death results, we call the deed manslaughter; when the assailant knew in advance the injury would be fatal, we call this deed murder. But when society places hundreds of proletarians in such a position that they inevitably meet a too early and unnatural death... and yet permits these conditions to remain, its deed is as surely murder as the deed of a single individual.

(1973 [1845]: 134)

For Marx and Engels, one of the consequences of the exploitation and poverty suffered by the proletariat was the preventable destruction of their health. For this, they held the capitalist system responsible.

While Marx may not have had all that much to say on the subject, subsequent Marxists have applied his ideas more systematically to the areas of health and health care. One of the major approaches taken by Marxists and those influenced by Marxist ideas has been to demonstrate that the inequalities generated by capitalist society cause those at the bottom of the social hierarchy to suffer more from disease than those at the top. The most famous piece of evidence to support this case is to be found in the *Black Report* (DHSS 1980), which was followed by *The Health Divide* (Whitehead 1988).

The Black Report was produced by a commission set up by the Labour government in the 1970s to examine the inequalities of health in Britain. Using government statistics that documented health according to five grades of occupational class, ranging from professional (class I) to unskilled workers (class V), the *Black Report* discovered that adult men in occupational class V had a mortality rate almost twice that of those in class I. Perhaps even more worrying was the fact that over time, instead of narrowing, this gap between the health of the well-off and the poor was widening. These findings were reinforced by the results of *The Health Divide*.

Marxist commentators have used the sort of information uncovered by Black and Whitehead to interrogate the underlying social tensions that lead to such inequalities. They have used the evidence of social inequalities in health to reinforce their claim that health and illness are largely determined by social and economic arrangements, and that capitalism's relentless pursuit of profit means that health for all is not possible within capitalist societies (Doyal 1979). Why should this be? What is it about capitalism that makes it inimical to health? At least three factors have been identified by Marxist commentators.

Exploitation and illness

First of all, it is argued that the exploitation of workers in the pursuit of profit inevitably leads to significant inequalities in the distribution of income. In turn, the distribution of health broadly mirrors the distribution of income, as the *Black Report* demonstrated. The reasons for this linkage are outlined by Doyal:

> In capitalist society income is a major determinant of the standard of housing individuals and families can obtain, of where they live, of their diet, and of their ability to remain warm and well clothed.
>
> (1979: 26)

One of the objections to this approach is that these inequalities can be explained by the poor habits of working class individuals, which leads them to tend to smoke and drink more than the well-off. This line of argument cuts little ice with Marxists:

> The dominant explanation of the greater ill health of people at the bottom of society focuses on individual behaviour. Ill health is seen as a personal responsibility. Socialists have taken a different view, pointing to the way companies put profit before health both in terms of what is produced and the way it is produced. We argue that the logic of capitalism is that it doesn't matter if junk food, cigarettes, alcohol or weapons can damage us as long as they sell. And it doesn't matter either, if workers in the factories or the people living near them are damaged by the way the product is made.
>
> (Mitchell 1984: 99)

This quotation from Mitchell indicates that Marxists do not restrict their critique of capitalism to the social inequalities that result from this form of economic organisation. Marxists are also interested in the health effects of both production and consumption. The physical processes of work are often dangerous and unhealthy. Workers may suffer directly, in the form of industrial injuries, or indirectly, for example through work-related stress.

Nor is it simply a matter of those directly involved in the production process. People are increasingly aware of the wider damage to the environment that is the byproduct of industrial production. From the perspective on consumption, Marxists argue that those commentators who concentrate on lifestyle factors in health ignore the huge pressures that capitalism puts on people to consume profit-making, but illness-inducing, products.

The political economy of AIDS and drug use

An interesting example of Marxist approaches to issues surrounding lifestyle and ill health can be found in recent anthropological research into the political economy of AIDS. This work is based upon the assumption that it is not an adequate response to blame AIDS upon the habits of its victims. The main point here is that rather than concentrating health prevention activities on the HIV risk behaviours of those groups within society at most risk of contracting AIDS, it is necessary to examine the broader social and economic contexts within which those behaviours take place (Glick Schiller 1992). For example, in a piece of research that was conducted in the mid-1970s before AIDS was recognised, Sharff (1987) argued that for many people, involvement in the drug trade was simply a matter of generating income for survival. She noted that one of the characteristics of mature capitalism was the division of the economy into primary and secondary sectors. The primary sector, which is highly technological, relies largely on a skilled and relatively well-paid labour force, which enjoys relatively secure working conditions. Conversely, the ever-growing secondary sector is labour intensive, relying on a transient and unskilled labour force. As a result, those who lie outside the primary labour market face the prospect of unemployment or low-paid work. Being in these economic positions, with their attendant lack of economic resources, means that people are required to engage in alternative market activities, one of these being the drug trade.

The effect of research such as Sharf's has been to encourage health care practitioners to widen their perspective on risk behaviour to include the social and economic context of that behaviour. Thus, for example, in an editorial in the *American Journal of Public Health*, it was stated that:

> It would be naive to conclude that we can radically change the course of
> the lives of individuals living in high-risk communities without addressing
> the issues of poverty, homelessness, and racism. The implementation of
> large-scale comprehensive prevention programs and more rational
> social policies can make incremental differences and improve the
> circumstances for some. That is sufficient reason to initiate immediate
> action. However, our nation will continue to be high-risk until we are
> willing to undertake the massive social and economic reforms that will
> equalize access to the opportunity structure.
>
> (Dryfoos 1991: 158)

The primary aim of this sort of approach is to get away from
regarding risk behaviour as an individual matter by placing it in
the socio-economic context in which it occurs. The logic of such
an approach is that if we concentrate simply on individuals, we are
only looking at the end product of a complex process. In order
fully to understand why people act in certain ways and, more
importantly, to minimise risky behaviour, we need to identify
those factors which encourage such behaviour. These factors are
often generated by the social and economic inequalities that result
from capitalism.

Recent research by Robert Carlson (1996), concentrating on
the relationship between AIDS and drug use, has taken the
Marxist approach to the AIDS epidemic even further. Carlson
argues that the sort of political economy approaches reviewed
above do not go far enough in that they tend to limit themselves
to the reform of capitalism, without examining the capitalist
worldview that lies at the basis of the unequal social relations that
pertain. Carlson returns to Marx's analysis of alienation, which, he
argues, involves a critique of capitalism not just as a kind of
economy, but also as a cosmology (a way of viewing the
universe). That cosmology 'is not attuned to the emergence of the
human potential, or what Marx referred to as "species being"'
(Carlson 1996: 272). According to Carlson, the fundamental
problem with the human condition under the capitalist
cosmology is that people regard themselves primarily as biologi-
cally separate entities, having little recognition of the connectedness between each other or between humanity and nature. Life is
regarded as a competition, a power struggle between individuals.
Furthermore, given the emphasis in capitalist society on the
production of profits through the sale of commodities, along with

the inevitable social inequalities and therefore unequal purchasing capacity that capitalism engenders, 'power is displayed by the ability to purchase commodities that symbolize success' (Carlson 1996: 271). From his ethnographic study of crack-cocaine users, Carlson concludes that:

> the crack-cocaine epidemic may be viewed as a terrifying reflection of what the myth of power taken to its extreme entails – that is, the fallacy that by consuming commodities and controlling others, meaningful relationships among individuals and broader domains can be created.
>
> (1996: 272)

Carlson observes that those in the disadvantaged ghettos of North America are stuck on the horns of a dilemma. On the one hand, they are bombarded with images of success. On the other hand, they know that they cannot aspire through legitimate means to the success that is displayed all around them. The use and peddling of crack provides an alternative route. By consuming crack, and experiencing its 'rush', people at least have the feeling of success and power. In a way, crack provides the ultimate commodity market. It engenders in its users an almost total individual self-centredness, in which commodity consumption takes precedence over moral values or social norms – people will do almost anything to obtain more crack. This elevates crack to a highly valuable commodity, bestowing enormous power on those who possess it. Thus, for example, Carlson notes that even small amounts of the drug, worth $5 or less, are enough to purchase the performance of sexual favours. This ability to control others to the extent of forcing them to perform terribly degrading acts 'raises the myth of power to previously unseen levels of self destruction' (Carlson 1996: 272). The central point that Carlson is trying to make here is that the crack-cocaine epidemic is not an aberration in capitalist society but rather a logical extension of the assumptions underlying the capitalist cosmology. It is, in short, a stark example of capitalism gone mad.

Capitalism and health care

Marxist critiques of capitalism and health have not been confined to the issue of how capitalism directly affects people's health.

Marxists have also examined how health care professions, most notably medicine, function for the benefit of capitalism. In doing so, they have been highly critical of the medical profession as it is currently constituted.

It is argued that, at a physical level, medicine aids the maintenance and reproduction of labour (Doyal 1979). In order to function, capitalism requires a reliable (and therefore healthy) workforce. This requirement has become even more important over time. In contrast to early industrialised societies, and contemporary developing societies, where labour is plentiful and expendable, the health of some sections of the labour force in highly technological societies has become very valuable to capitalism. The more sophisticated technology gets, the more complex it becomes, which means that those who work with it need to be highly skilled. It takes a lot of time and money to train people to the skill levels often required by modern technology. The cost to capital through the loss of skilled labour is therefore very high, so it is important to capitalism that skilled labourers remain as healthy as possible. Of course, those in professional and skilled jobs only make up one section of the workforce. It might be argued that the rise of private health care insurance among these groups, with a corresponding squeeze of public health care provisions on which other, less well-off groups rely, is an indication of how health care is becoming differentiated on the grounds of people's positions within the capitalist system.

Marxists also argue that medicine, through its control of childbirth, plays an important role in regulating human (and therefore labour) reproduction. Once again, the fact that Western societies no longer require a huge, unskilled labour force, but a smaller, healthier one, can be posited as one explanation of medicine's increasing interventions into the area of birth control (Doyal 1979).

One of the problems with these sorts of argument is that they can be applied to almost any social system of which one cares to think. Any society, whether capitalist or not, requires people to be sufficiently healthy in order to be able to produce those goods and services which society requires. It is therefore rather unfair to single out capitalism and blame it for doing something that even communist societies would have to do. The Marxist response to this objection points to inequalities in the provision of care.

Despite the introduction of nationalised health, different groups of people enjoy different levels of health care. This sort of inequality is not simply about being able to afford private health insurance. Even when being treated by the same doctors, working class people tend to receive an inferior service. A study by Cartwright and O'Brien (1976) compared the treatment of working class and middle class patients by GPs. They discovered that the time GPs spent in consultation with working class patients was considerably less than that spent with middle class patients, that they gave working class patients less information and that they knew them less well.

Another objection to the Marxist claim that medicine is simply used by capitalism to maintain and reproduce the labour force is that medicine does not provide value for money. Health care systems in advanced capitalist countries suck up a huge proportion of wealth. Given the evidence that medicine has not really made that great a difference to the health of populations (McKeown 1976), and given Marxists' claims about the profit motivation of capitalists, such expenditure is difficult to understand.

The Marxist response to this point is that, in addition to the material role that medicine plays, it also plays an ideological role, influencing the ways in which people think about capitalism. Navarro (1976) argues that the way in which medicine approaches health and illness supports capitalism by influencing our attitudes. Here, we can see how Navarro is adopting Marx's (1970) argument that the intellectual stances adopted within a society are merely part of the social superstructure that is founded upon the base of economic relations.

First of all, medicine tends to concentrate on the individual rather than the social origins of disease. Illness is seen as the result either of individual misfortune, such as succumbing to infection, or as a matter of individual responsibility, such as contracting lung cancer as a consequence of cigarette smoking. This approach plays down the importance of the various social and economic factors discussed in the previous section, which militate towards ill health. This individualistic approach is reinforced by medicine's concentration on curative rather than preventative health care. By concentrating on cures of illnesses with which people have already been stricken, medicine once again fails properly to address the social and economic causes of disease, thus, Marxists argue, masking the unhealthy nature of much capitalist production. In short, medicine is regarded as creating a smokescreen that hides the extent to which capitalism is responsible for both the physical and mental ills of the population.

Second, medical care is seen as providing capitalism with a valuable public relations image. Universal health care gives capitalism the image of being caring, once again masking other facets of the capitalist system that are actually bad for health. Moreover, much-trumpeted advances in medical science make capitalism look progressive, creating the illusion that some time in the future, through ever improved technology, capitalism will be able to solve the problems of health and illness once and for all.

Finally, the authoritarian and hierarchical way in which doctors treat their patients – especially their working class, female and black patients, reinforces the hierarchies of capitalist society:

> The idea that it is only the doctor who can cure, and the belief that one's mind and body can be separated and treated according to the laws of science, both serve to emphasise the loss of individual autonomy and the feelings of powerlessness so common in other areas of social and economic life. People come to believe that they have little control over their own bodies, just as, for example, they have so little control over the conditions in which they spend their working lives.
>
> (Doyal 1979: 43)

To summarise, the basic Marxist argument in relation to health care is that the way in which it is organised within capitalist society means that it mirrors and reinforces the relations of inequality that are at the core of capitalism.

Medicine and imperialism

Probably the starkest example of medicine's oppressive role within capitalism can be found in its collaboration in a particular form of capitalism – imperialism. In using the term 'imperialism', Marxists are referring to the expansion of capitalist states and economies into other areas of the world. As Paul (1978) points out:

> Imperialism is an excellent vantage point from which to see the social and political functions of medicine. In the impoverishment, plunder, and violence of the colonies and neocolonies, capitalist social relations

assume their most transparent and clearly identifiable image. Medicine has from the beginning functioned in the service of imperialism, supporting logically the voracious search for ever wider markets and profitable deals.

(Paul 1978: 271–2)

Using the example of the French take-over of Morocco in the nineteenth and early twentieth centuries, Paul works through the various functions that medicine served for France's imperial intentions. The first of these involved doctors acting as covert diplomats. Here, doctors, using their professional skills, insinuated themselves into the favour of the domestic élites. Taking advantage of their capacity to cure and the cloak of professional confidence, they managed to establish positions of contact where more traditional diplomatic efforts had failed. Using (or rather, abusing) their position, they were able to argue for favourable terms for treaties, contracts for business, banks and mining companies, as well as to gain intelligence and to sow discord when this suited the purposes of France. Thus, for example, a certain Dr Linarès was the principle diplomatic figure in the Moroccan court for over a quarter of a century. His achievements were summed up by one French ambassador, who described him as a 'precious liaison with the [government], capable of neutralizing rival influences... and preparing the way for what is called "the peaceful penetration" of Morocco' (quoted in Paul 1978: 275). Nor was Linarès the only physician to take on such a role – scores of doctors were prepared to subsume their medical responsibilities to the requirements of French imperialism.

Medical practitioners did not confine their efforts to the Moroccan élite. Using the cover of their professional role, they were also involved as spies and propagandists among the Moroccan masses. For example, the French army set up mobile medical units that acted as the vanguard for the invasion of 1907. These units were sent out into the countryside to 'care' for the members of local tribes. Using the occasion of medical consultations, they came into contact with local leaders. At this point, they offered the leaders a choice – the continuance of the sort of benevolent care that they were offering or the prospect of certain death and destruction if they attempted to resist the might of the French army. By such means, the French imperialist forces won numerous victories without actually having to do battle. Army physicians were also attached to intelligence operations, offering medical care in exchange for militarily useful information.

Medicine was also used as a powerful propaganda tool in France itself, persuading the French populace of the worthiness of imperial expansion into Morocco. Before invasion, European physicians lobbied in favour of colonial take-over. They described the poor conditions of health in Morocco and argued that the introduction of Western medicine would lead to great improvements. Medicine reinforced the view of Moroccans as being ignorant savages, unable to look after their own health. The French government was then able to use the Moroccan 'need' for Western health care as a justification for their invasion. Throughout the period of imperial occupation, the colonialists continued to use medical accomplishments as a powerful excuse for their actions.

It should be noted that this sort of relationship between medicine and imperialism is confined neither to France nor to the period of initial colonial expansion. Paul (1978) also cites the case of the USA's invasion of Vietnam. Once again, there is considerable evidence that American physicians prostituted their professional responsibilities for the cause of America. Thus, for example, in 1967 President Johnson commissioned a distinguished team of American physicians, which included the vice-president of the American Medical Association, to investigate health conditions in Vietnam. Among other strange findings, the team concluded that the widespread petroleum burns suffered by the civilian populace were not caused by the blanket napalm bombing in which the US air force was engaging but rather the 'careless use of gasoline in stoves not intended for this purpose' (quoted by Paul 1978: 279).

There are also occasions when physicians have become directly involved in the barbarities of imperialism. A stark example of this is provided by the Martiniquean psychiatrist and anti-imperialist activist, Franz Fanon. Fanon (1978), who was involved in the Algerian Revolution against French occupation (1954–62), graphically describes the role of physicians in the counter-revolution. The most horrific aspect of this account is probably the involvement of doctors in torture and interrogation processes. Thus, for example, physicians frequently administered 'truth serums', the aim of which was to induce loss of control and a blunting of consciousness and thus decrease resistance to interrogation. Administration of these intravenous drugs was often carried out repeatedly over several days. When the survivors of this practice came to be treated by Fanon and his colleagues, they were typically suffering from:

> a certain inability to distinguish the true from the false, and an almost obsessive fear of saying what should remain hidden. We must always remember that there is hardly an Algerian who is not a party to at least one secret of the revolution. Months after this torture, the former prisoner hesitates to say his name, the town where he was born. Every question is first experienced as a repetition of the torturer–tortured relationship.

> (Fanon 1978: 243–4)

Even more alarming were those psychiatrists who were prepared to administer electric shock treatments to prisoners and then to question them during the waking phase. Those who were lucky enough to survive these interrogations (and many did not) were severely mentally disturbed. As Fanon puts it, 'what is brought to us is a personality in shreds' (1978: 244).

Doctors were also employed in torture centres in order to keep prisoners sufficiently healthy to be reinterrogated:

> Under the circumstances, the most important thing is for the prisoner not to give the slip to the team in charge of the questioning: in other words, to remain alive. Everything – heart stimulants, massive doses of vitamins – is used before, during and after the sessions to keep the Algerian hovering between life and death. Ten times the doctor intervenes, ten times he gives the prisoner back to the pack of torturers.

> (Fanon 1978: 244)

Fanon also accused physicians of collaborating with torturers by providing death certificates citing natural causes for death when in fact death was due to torture or summary execution.

These are horrific tales and involve a very dark picture of the role of physicians. The purpose of recounting them is not to give the impression that all doctors are somehow potential torturers or apologists for colonialists. Fanon himself was a physician who used his skills to ameliorate the dire effects that the French military had upon the health of the Algerian people. The point of this section has been to illustrate the Marxist argument that medicine does not function outside the social relations within which it operates. Marxists argue that where those social relations are oppressive, there will be often found doctors, who after all usually enjoy social and economic privilege within those societies, who will be prepared to use their professional skills in maintaining them.

Making profits from illness

The third strand of Marxist critiques of capitalism in relation to health concentrates on the way in which capitalism has turned the maintenance and recovery of health into a profit-making commodity. One of the major targets of this attack has been what is termed the transnational pharmaceutical industry. This industry is one of the most successful and powerful sectors of the capitalist economy. Its stature is reflected in the fact that, in 1994, its annual sales amounted to $256 billion, more than the total health expenditure of the 'developing' world and Eastern Europe combined. A single drug – Zantac – used to treat gastric ulcers, earned Glaxo Wellcome $3.6 billion: more than the gross national product of Jamaica (Chetley 1995). Companies such as Glaxo Wellcome have become so large and powerful that they are now global organisations no longer beholden to any nation state (Tucker 1996); it is for this reason that they are described as 'transnational'.

It might be argued that there is nothing wrong with a large global volume of drug sales – quite the contrary, in that it indicates that sophisticated medical interventions are now enjoyed by the vast majority of people living on the planet. However, the Marxist response to this is that the vast majority of the drugs generating the huge incomes that the transnational pharmaceutical industry enjoys are of little value. There are approximately 100,000 different drugs on the market. However, this figure hides a lack of diversity in that many of these are 'me too' drugs, which involve only minor chemical changes to existing products but which are eligible for a new patent, thus protecting the monopolisation of profits (Tucker 1996). There is considerable evidence that the vast majority of this plethora of 'new' drugs have not contributed to an improvement in pharmaceutical interventions in ill health. For example, a 7-year survey of new drugs by the US Food and Drugs Administration found that only 3 per cent made 'an important potential contribution to existing therapies; 13 per cent made a 'modest potential contribution', while 84 per cent made 'little or no potential contribution' (quoted in Chetley 1995: 22). Similarly, the World Health Organisation (WHO) states that two-thirds of all drugs used by children may be of little or no use (Rylance 1987).

Much of the efforts of the transnational pharmaceuticals to sell their wares are concentrated on the developing world, where they spend between 20 and 30 per cent of their sales on promotion and advertising (Chetley 1990). Thus, for example, while in Britain there is one drugs company representative to every 20 doctors, the figure for the Philippines is one for every two doctors (Melrose 1993).

That profits come before health for the transnational pharmaceutical industry was starkly demonstrated by its response to the WHO's ethical marketing code. The code included restrictions on the marketing of breast milk substitutes, which had been identified as promoting malnutrition in children because, after being hooked on substitutes, many mothers were unable to afford the product and were also unable to return to breast feeding. The International Federation of Pharmaceutical Manufacturers Associations challenged the code, marshalling the backing of the US government. The US delegate to the WHO was quite candid about the reasons as to why the USA was prepared to vote against the marketing code:

> I think that most delegates know that the United States was the only country to vote against the adoption of the breast milk substitutes marketing code in 1981. Before then and ever since, it has been our strong position that the World Health Organisation should not be involved in efforts to regulate or control the commercial practices of private industry, even when the products may relate to concerns about health.
>
> (quoted in Hardon *et al*. 1992: 59)

A similar campaign was mounted by the industry against the WHO's essential drugs policy, in which the WHO advocated that the number of drugs used in national health programmes should be restricted to between 200 and 250 in order to reduce drugs bills and to ensure that only essential drugs were prescribed. Although the industry eventually accepted the code, they continue to insist that it is not relevant to developed countries (Tucker 1996).

Marxists conclude from evidence like this that health care industries such as the pharmaceutical industry are not really interested in health but are simply one very powerful component of the capitalist economic structure, the purpose of which is to generate profits. Moreover, they argue that as long as the health care industry is organised in a capitalist fashion, this will remain the case, given that the *raison d'être* of capitalist industry is to maximise profit. From this, they conclude that the capitalist organisation of health care is inimicable to the promotion of health. For Marxists, it will only be when health care industries are brought under social control that there will be any guarantee that they will truly engage in the role they pretend to play, namely the improvement of the health of the population.

Nursing example: Marxism and informal care

Marxism has, to date, not had a great deal of influence upon nursing literature concerning practice. One exception, however, is Jacqueline Bridges and Judith Lynam's 'Informal carers: a Marxist analysis of social, political, and economic forces underpinning the role' (1993). In their article, Bridges and Lynam note that while nursing theories acknowledge the importance of the environment, including the social environment, to health, they continue to maintain a highly individualistic approach, treating the environment as an immutable force to which people must adapt rather than something that can be altered as a result of nursing intervention. However, following McMurray (1991), they note that if nursing concepts such as advocacy are to be properly implemented, advocacy needs to be widened to include the social, political and economic circumstances of clients. On these grounds, they argue that Marxism, which by definition addresses these areas of social life, can contribute to a useful expansion of the domain of nursing.

Using the example of the rise of informal care of the elderly, Bridges and Lynam work through the various stages whereby the logic of capitalism affects the everyday lives of informal carers. They start their analysis at the level of the capitalist élite, with its imperative to maximise profit. One of the most significant drains on profit potential involves its siphoning off in the form of public expenditure. It is therefore in the interests of the capitalist economic sector to ensure that public expenditure is kept to a minimum. As a result, there is pressure upon governments in capitalist societies to keep down their costs. Bridges and Lynam argue this is reflected in the move away from expensive state-funded institutional care for the elderly towards community care, which relies heavily on unpaid informal labour. In addition, they note the patriarchal nature of capitalist society, which is in this case reflected in the reliance upon women as unpaid carers. Thus, their argument is that at the next level of capitalist society, that of government, legislative policies promoting informal care are reflections of capital's economic need to maximise profits and its ideological commitment to male-dominated hierarchies. Once again, we return to Marx's (1970) analysis of the relationship between the economic base and the political and ideological superstructure.

The next level in the capitalist chain is that of bureaucracy. Once again, this is highly influenced by the previous level, that of government, in that the programmes devised by those charged with administering the care of the elderly are:

> most likely to be maintained or expanded [if they] receive government support in the form of financial support or policy support. A successful program, therefore, is one that reflects government ideology. Bureaucrats thus have a vested interest in reproducing ruling class ideology, as the success of their programs will reinforce their current position in the power structure.
>
> (Bridges and Lynam 1993: 41)

Next down the line in the capitalist hierarchy come what Bridges and Lynam term 'the producers', a group that consists of health care practitioners. Once again, Bridges and Lynam argue that practitioners have vested interests in collaborating with the capitalist construction of health care:

> producers translate ruling class ideology into practice through cooperation with programs set at an administrative level and the use of priorities predetermined by the government and the bureaucrats. Producers' interests in maximising personal profits and retaining current structural position are served by translating ruling class ideology into practice.
>
> (1993: 43)

The significance of this level of the capitalist hierarchy is that, at this point, ideology becomes reality, but it is also at this point that consumers can articulate their true needs in the face of that realisation of ideology. Given that carers tend to be disadvantaged and unsupported within the economic and social circumstances currently pertaining, there is likely to be a gulf between the needs of the carer and the ideology of the ruling class. Here we come to nurses' dilemma of whether to act as an advocate, promoting the needs and desires of their clients, or to act in the interests of the bureaucracy for which they work. Nurses are thus faced with a choice: do they legitimate ruling class ideology through co-operation with programmes legislated for by government and devised by bureaucracies or do they side with the client by attempting to challenge the structure with which they are faced? In the former case, the practitioner treats the circumstances of the informal carer as immutable and concentrates her action on providing some assistance to the carer in coping with those circumstances, so that informal care can continue. In the latter case, the practitioner challenges the supposed immutability of social circumstances and contemplates alternatives, asking such questions as:

> How could care be shared more equally among family members? How could other resources for informal care in the community be mobilized? How could the state offer sufficient alternatives for care to ensure that the family member has a choice in whether to provide care? Are there other options to care, such as participation in the labor market, open to the carer?
>
> (Bridges and Lynam 1993: 43–4)

Asking such questions is all well and good, but how should health care practitioners and informal carers go about getting them answered to their satisfaction? Bridges and Lynam suggest a number of avenues in which nurses can involve themselves. These include helping consumers to articulate their needs, helping to organise carers, working with community groups and working at the level of professional organisations to effect change. However, the problem that many Marxist analysts would have with this sort of approach is that it is 'reformist': it seeks to reform the system rather than radically change it. Thus, Bridges and Lynam argue that the collective mobilisation of nurses and clients would pose a significant threat to the existing power structure, concluding that

'To retain their elected structural position, the ruling class would be forced to rethink their ideologies and strategies in favor of the consumer' (1993: 44). For orthodox Marxism, this is to lay too much emphasis upon political institutions and to ignore the economic relations on which those institutions are based. From such a viewpoint, politicians are at best only part of the ruling class, which fundamentally consists of those who own and control the means of production. As Marx himself put it, 'political power is precisely the official expression of antagonism in civil society' (1974 [1847]: 197). Thus the oppressive nature of the state is merely a symptom of underlying conflict that is associated with unequal economic distribution. This is not to deny that significant struggles and changes take place in the political realm but rather to assert that a deeper analysis is needed to understand why politicians adopt the positions that they do.

Irrespective of the degree of power and autonomy we ascribe to the state, it remains the case that Bridges and Lynam's work provides a passionate argument that the scope of nursing practice should not be confined to individual issues. Since what happens to people as individuals depends to a considerable degree upon the political, social and economic circumstances in which they find themselves, it follows that nursing care, if it is to aspire to holism, must take account of those circumstances. This may mean that nursing will come into conflict with the powers that be, especially when their clients are situated in economically disadvantaged positions in society. Bridges and Lynam's challenge to nurses is to take their caring responsibilities seriously and face up to the need to respond effectively to health problems that are generated by an unequal society.

Recommended further reading

There are a considerable number of books that provide selections of Marx's writings. A short and accessible tour through his vast output can be found in Bottomore and Rubel's *Karl Marx: Selected Writings in Sociology and Social Philosophy* (1966). As far as Marxist approaches to health care are concerned, Lesley Doyal's *The Political Economy of Health* (1979), although now rather dated, provides the most comprehensive Marxist treatment.

4 Weber and professional closure

Introduction

The final member of the generally accepted founding triumvirate of the discipline of sociology, along with Marx and Durkheim, was Max Weber (1864–1920). Despite being prevented from working for long periods by depression, Weber's output and range of interests was staggering. In addition to sociology, he made contributions to law, economics and history. His areas of interest within sociology included methodology, the comparative study of religion, the rise of the ethos of rationality and its relationship to the development of capitalism, and the studies of bureaucracy and social stratification. In all these areas, his ideas continue to exert a huge influence on contemporary sociological thought.

The problem for a textbook such as this is that there is not enough space to include discussion of all these areas or even of all those areas that may be of relevance to nursing, which include his promotion of qualitative methodology, his analysis of rationality, his study of bureaucracies and his conceptualisation of stratification. Of these, I have chosen to concentrate on the latter in this chapter, partly because his approach to stratification was a response to Marx and therefore fits well with the previous chapter, but more importantly because Weber's work on stratification has fostered a sociological approach to the professions that is highly appropriate to the occupation of nursing. In relation to his qualitative methodology, a discussion of this will be included in Chapter 6, on the grounds that Weber was a seminal figure in the development of social phenomenology. Similarly, his analysis of the rise of Western rationality will be discussed in Chapter 7, on the grounds that it helped to lay the basis for critical theory's critique of capitalism. As for bureaucracy, despite its salience to nursing in terms of the highly bureaucratic nature of health care institutions, I am afraid it must be left for another day.

As usual, this chapter is shaped like a funnel. It starts with a discussion of Weber's general theory of stratification and then moves on to the specific area of social closure, a mechanism used by groups to improve their standing in society. The chapter then moves to those neo-Weberian scholars that have used his ideas on social closure to analyse the position of professions in modern society. (These scholars are called neo-Weberian because although they use Weber's ideas as fruitful sources, they are far from being disciples who are prepared to accept his word as gospel.) Finally, I include two nursing examples that relate social closure to the occupation of nursing, namely Anne Witz's (1992) discussion of the registration campaign at the turn of this century and my own analysis of the effects of strategies of social closure upon the everyday work of clinical nurses (Porter 1995b).

Class, status and party

One of the classical, and perhaps overworked, controversies within social theory involves the differences between Marx's construction of class and Max Weber's notion of social stratification. It will be remembered from the previous chapter that at the core of Marx's analysis of the social world was his identification of the fundamental division between those who owned and controlled the means of production and those who did not. Within capitalism, this division was between the bourgeoisie and the proletariat. In short, for Marx the fundamental tension in society lay in the economic arrangements pertaining.

Weber's response to the Marxist view of divisions within society was to argue that Marx was only partially right in his diagnosis. He did so on the grounds that class differences entailed only one of the divisions that distinguished groups within society. Classes are formed out of the placing of groups within what he termed the 'economic order' (Weber 1970 [1922]: 194). However, Weber argued that there were another two fundamental divisions between social groups that had no necessary relationship to the class position of those groups. The first of these divisions occurred in what he termed the 'social order'. This involved competition between groups for social honour and prestige. The final division occurred within the 'legal order' and entailed the struggle for political power. Thus, Weber argued that a comprehensive view of the dynamics of social division should involve an examination of three different categories: class, status and party. I shall briefly expand on each of these conceptions in turn.

Class

Weber is very specific in his definition of class, arguing that there are three criteria that require to be satisfied before we can talk of a group being a class:

> (1) a number of people have in common a specific causal component of their life chances, in so far as (2) this component is represented exclusively by economic interests in the possession of goods and opportunities for income, and (3) is represented under the conditions of the commodity or labor markets.
>
> (1970: 181)

This definition requires some unpacking. In relation to (1), Weber is arguing that the first criterion for the existence of a class is that there should exist a group of people whose circumstances lead them to have a similar access to 'life chances', life chances being defined as the capacity to acquire goods and services, the external living conditions enjoyed and the quality of personal life experiences. However this is, for Weber, too general a definition. As I have already noted, he places classes into the specific area of the economic order. This is the point that he is making in (2): class divisions relate only to differences in life chances in so far as those life chances are affected by economic considerations. Put another way, class relates to the degree of economic power that different groups have to access the good life. The final part of Weber's definition – (3) – relates the conditions under which economic power is distributed. Unlike Marx, who sees classes as being constituted by the great binary struggle between the owners and controllers and the non-owners and non-controllers of productive property, Weber sees economic struggle as being a far more diverse process, involving a plurality of groups all competing with each other in the market, where goods and services are exchanged for a price. He concedes that the ownership of property confers great advantage upon one's position in the market, and that '"Property" and "lack of property" are, therefore, the basic categories of all class situations' (1970: 182). However, within these categories, there is a huge amount of differentiation. So, for example, among those with property, there may be a class of entrepreneurs and a class of agricultural owners, each with their different and perhaps competing interests. Conversely, those who lack property will be differentiated according to the services that they provide. Their economic success will depend on the market value of their services – the price that the market will bear for those services. Thus for Weber, '"Class situation" is... ultimately "market situation"' (1970: 182). This is an important point to which we will return later.

Status

As I have already noted, as well as class differences, Weber also argued that there were differences within the social order. In other words, groups in society are not just differentiated according to their place in the market; there are also divisions of status:

> In contrast to the purely economically determined 'class situation' we wish to designate as 'status situation' every typical component of the life fate of men that is determined by a specific, positive or negative, social estimation of *honor*.
>
> (Weber 1970: 186–7)

While there is often a linkage between class and status, with, for example, the economically powerful also enjoying social status, this is not always the case. Think, for example, of the 1980s yuppies, young men and women who often made large fortunes from their activities in the money markets and other such institutions. While these people where economically very successful, they were also seen as *nouveau riche* upstarts who indulged in a gauche and profligate lifestyle. In other words, their economic success brought them little social honour. Conversely, we might think of nurses. No-one could accuse this occupational group of spectacular economic success, yet nurses are accorded a considerable degree of honour and respect in society as a result of social perceptions about their caring selflessness (do you recognise yourself here?).

In one way, nurses are an exception to the status rule in that, as Weber points out, status stratification often goes hand in hand with the monopolisation of goods and services. Thus, for example, an honorific group may have a monopoly over wearing a certain costume or the right to bear arms. What differentiates these groups from economically privileged groups is that they are stratified not according to the production of goods but according to their consumption of goods. In other words, it is their exclusive style of life that marks them out. The cynic might point out here that it is only those groups who have succeeded economically who will have the wherewithal to consume certain goods to which their fellow humans cannot gain access.

How do status groups differentiate themselves from other groups? Weber argues that there are a number of ways in which this happens. These range from fairly loose social conventions, such as the adherence to certain sartorial fashions such as Armani suits, through to very rigid divisions, such as occurs in the caste system in India, whereby a person is born into a caste to which she will belong for life.

As I have already noted, Weber concedes that classes and status groups frequently overlap. Thus, for example, an occupational group may be seen as a class because it will enjoy a certain market position by dint of the relationship between supply and demand for the goods or services it provides. However, it can also be seen as a status group because 'normally, it successfully claims social honor only by virtue of the special style of life which may be determined by it' (Weber 1970: 193). Once again, this is a pertinent point to which we will return later.

Party

The third and final division in society identified by Weber is that of 'parties'. Parties, for Weber, are groups who have a specific agenda, and their aim is to gain social power in order to achieve the goals identified in that agenda. As Weber puts it, parties live in a house of power. They use a variety of means, ranging from naked violence through to parliamentary cunning, to attain social power. While they are usually at least partly associated with certain classes and/or status groups, parties may also be independent.

Education and social closure

In common with the usual format of chapters in this book, we have thus far been discussing a very general aspect of Weber's sociological theory, which may at first appear to have little pertinence to nursing issues. However, I hope it will soon become clear how Weber's notions of the relationship between class and status might have some bearing on discussions about the profession of nursing. However, before we get that specific, there are a number of other stages through which we need to go. The first is Weber's identification of the process of social closure and how this relates to the acquisition of educational credentials.

Weber (1968a [1922]) used the term 'social closure' to describe the mechanism whereby social collectivities, be they classes or status groups, attempt to close off from other groups' access to resources and advantages. For Weber, social closure involves the arbitrary identification of a certain attribute and its subsequent use as a criterion for eligibility to be part of that group. The criterion might be based on a characteristic of external competitors, such as their race, religion or social origin, or it may be based on 'shared qualities *acquired* through upbringing, apprenticeship and training' of the members of the group itself (1968a: 344). It is in the operation of the latter-type social closure that educational credentials have their importance. Weber (1968b [1922]) identifies the prestige of what he calls the 'patent of education', acquired through specialist examinations. However, it is more than simply a matter of social honour, given that 'this prestige can again be turned to economic advantage' (1968b: 1000). Thus, educational credentials can be used to enhance both the status and class situation of those who gain them. Here we can begin to see the importance of Weber's observation mentioned earlier that class and status positions can overlap and reinforce each other.

Weber takes a very cynical line on the reason for the ever-increasing emphasis on education in Western societies, refusing to accept that it is simply a matter of a thirst for knowledge:

> The elaboration of the diplomas from universities, business and engineering colleges, and the universal clamor for the creation of further educational certificates in all fields serve the formation of a privileged

stratum in bureaus and in offices. Such certificates support their holders' claims for connubium [intermarriage] with the notables... claims to be admitted into the circles that adhere to 'codes of honor,' claims for a 'status-appropriate' salary instead of a wage according to performance... and, above all, claims to the monopolization of socially and economically advantageous positions. If we hear from all sides demands for the introduction of regulated curricula culminating in specialized examinations, the reason behind this is, of course, not a suddenly awakened 'thirst for education,' but rather the desire to limit the supply of candidates for these positions and to monopolize them for the holders of educational patents. For such monopolization, the 'examination' is today the universal instrument – hence its irresistible advance,

(Weber 1968b: 1000)

From this sort of critique of the self-serving motives behind educational patents, it is not a big step to apply Weber's analysis to those social groups whose status and class position rely most heavily upon their possession of such patents, namely the professions. It is to neo-Weberian treatments of the professions that we will now turn.

The social closure of professions

Weber's basic theoretical construct has provided fertile soil for those sociologists seeking to understand the economic power and social prestige that is enjoyed by professional groups such as medicine. The basic line of argument taken by neo-Weberian analysts of the professions is that these occupational groups have managed to attain a privileged position both economically and in terms of status. In relation to economic power, they have succeeded in monopolising market supply through social closure, specifically by using specialist examinations and exclusive registration based on attainment of those examinations. Having attained a monopoly, they have also succeeded in restricting the supply of their services, which has had the effect of pushing up the prices they can charge. In terms of status, social closure, combined with a claim to such attributes as altruism and ethicality, has had the effect of giving them a position of honour within society. To put bones on this thesis, I will briefly review the ideas of three neo-Weberian critics of the professions, putting specific emphasis on the profession of medicine.

Berlant and professional monopoly

Basing his work on Weber's notion of monopolisation (the process whereby groups gain exclusive control over goods, services or market position), Berlant (1975) identified ten aspects of monopolisation that are applicable to the historical development of the classic professions of medicine and law in Britain and America. I include a number of them here, showing in brackets how each characteristic of monopolisation might be reflected in the characteristics of the medical profession. Aspects of monopolisation include: the separation of the performance of services from the satisfaction of client interests ('doctor knows best' – it is the prerogative of the doctor, rather than the patient, to diagnose what is wrong with the patient and to prescribe the most appropriate treatment); the creation of scarcity (often through a restriction of the number of physicians trained, which has the effect of reducing the supply of medical expertise); the monopolisation of supply (only registered medical practitioners are able to diagnose illness and prescribe certain drugs); the restriction of group membership by means of social closure (achieved through the registration of eligible practitioners); the elimination of external competition (as is evidenced in the historical sidelining of midwifery by obstetrics); and the development of group solidarity and co-operativeness (have you ever seen a situation in which an individual doctor comes under suspicion of committing an error and her colleagues close ranks to protect her? Come to think of it, have you ever compared her colleagues' responses to the responses of a nurse's colleagues in the same sort of situation?).

Johnson and professional power

A similar critique of the established professions has been made by Terence Johnson (1972), who argues that professions attain their powerful position through the use of at least three strategies. Johnson starts by observing that the prices of services within the market are almost impossible to determine according to their intrinsic value – can we put a price on a bed bath or the cleaning of a leg ulcer that can be justified in their own terms, irrespective of the circumstances in which they occur? Because the price of such services cannot be determined according to their intrinsic nature, they are socially determined. As a result, the power relationship between consumers and producers is of paramount importance. Groups that are able attain high prices for their services do so by attaining a powerful market situation, in which their requirements in relation to price take precedence over the requirements of those who consume their services.

The fundamental mechanisms of the market are supply and demand. Because high supply or low demand means that there are more goods or services on offer than people really want, they will lower prices. Conversely, low supply and/or high demand, because they involve a situation in which there are not enough goods and services to go around, lead those who want them to compete for them, thus increasing price. Johnson notes that, reflecting these market laws, the first strategy used by professions involves a minimisation of supply by means of restriction of entry into their occupation. This means that there will never be enough professionals to satisfy the demands of clients for their services. Think, for example, of surgical waiting lists that result from there not being enough surgeons. Professions are able to restrict entry through control over training and the qualifications required for membership. It might be noted that the success of occupations such as medicine in manipulating the market in their favour is a prime example of Weber's observation that class position is essentially market position.

The second strategy used by professionals to attain and maintain the power they enjoy is what Johnson terms 'the promotion of occupational homogeneity'. The aim here is to prevent members of the occupation from entering into open competition and conflict with each other, thus challenging the monopoly that they have attained as a group. Professional control over the content of training, including the hidden curriculum, along with common rituals and occupational jargon, encourage a common outlook. In addition, such homogeneity is maintained through the myth of equal competence (often supported by restrictions on individual advertising) whereby physicians, for example, go to great pains, in the face of overwhelming lay scepticism, to assert that one will get the same quality of treatment, irrespective of by whom one is being treated. The justification for such an assertion lies in the claim that all physicians have successfully completed specialist examinations ensuring that they have reached a high level of competence.

The third strategy discussed by Johnson refers to the status enjoyed by professionals. He argues that the minimisation of supply and the maintenance of monopoly are reinforced by the favourable image that professions are able to project of themselves and the services they provide. Not only do they promote an image of altruism and ethicality, as I have already mentioned, but they also assert that these claims should be judged internally. When physicians are accused of breaking the ethical codes by which they are expected to abide, they are not usually brought to task by means of the general legal system; rather, they are judged by their peers through the mechanism of their professional registering body. As a result, all but the most lurid cases are kept from the public eye. The favourable image of professionals is also reinforced by their claims to the skills that they possess. They argue that the high financial rewards they receive is not simply a result of the useful work they do (after all, refuse disposal workers engage in work that is indispensable to the well-being of urban societies, but they receive only a fraction of a surgeon's wage), but also because of the complex skills they possess and the long period of time taken in training to attain those skills.

To summarise Johnson's argument, the importance of market control, homogeneity and image-building means that professionalism 'becomes redefined as a particular type of occupational control rather than an expression of the inherent nature of particular occupations' (Johnson 1972: 45).

Freidson and professional autonomy

It will be seen from the discussion thus far that neo-Weberians are rather sceptical about the claims professions make for themselves. This theme of scepticism is repeated in the work of Eliot Freidson, who challenged some of the rather credulous approaches that previous sociologists had taken towards the professions. It will be remembered, for example, from Chapter 2, how Talcott Parsons (1951) identified what he saw as the pattern variables of the medical role, attributing to physicians affective neutrality, universalism, achievement orientation, role specificity and collective orientation. Parsons was not the only one at the time to take such a benign approach. A group of sociologists known as trait theorists spent much time and effort trying to work out just what were the characteristics that distinguished professions from other, common or garden occupations. This all started with Flexner's (1915) list of six criteria, which regarded professional activity as intellectual, learned, practical, taught, internally organised and motivated by altruism. Since then, there have been numerous attempts to define professions, such as that by Carr-Saunders and Wilson, who argued that 'The application of an intellectual technique to the ordinary business of life, acquired as a result of prolonged and specialized training, is the chief distinguishing characteristic of a profession' (1933: 491). The problem with such attempts is that they all tend to come up with different lists of criteria. Thus, Millerson (1964), in an extensive review of trait theory literature that looked at the work of 21 authors, came up with no less than 23 'essential' professional attributes. None of these attributes was accepted as essential by all the authors reviewed. Indeed, nine of them were identified by only one author each.

It was in relation to this background that Freidson attempted to redefine the essential nature of professions from a less credulous standpoint. For Freidson, the one trait that can be attached to professions is their success in gaining a privileged market position by means of state sponsorship. This privileged position means that they have a high degree of autonomy over their practice:

> the most strategic difference [that separates professions from other occupations] lies in legitimate, organized autonomy – that a profession is distinct from other occupations in that it has been given the right to control its own work... Unlike other occupations, professions are *deliberately* granted autonomy, including the exclusive right to determine who can legitimately do its work and how the work should be done.
>
> (1970: 71–2)

Essentially, Freidson provides us with a variation on the Weberian theme that the actions of occupational groups are not essentially motivated by higher concerns but are in fact highly self-interested. It is on these grounds that Freidson rejects definitions of professions in terms of their education or their altruism, in favour of his identification of autonomy as being their core attribute. This autonomy, in turn, provides professionals with an extremely powerful market position, in that they are not beholden to clients, as are most occupations, for their actions or for the prices that they set for those actions.

Dual closure strategies

Thus far, we have been looking at how Weber's theories of social closure and monopolisation might be used to examine the privileged market and status position of the classical professions, notably medicine. What I now wish to turn to are those occupations, such as nursing, which have had some difficulty in breaking into this charmed circle. However, before doing so, it is necessary to address the influential work of Frank Parkin (1979), who has expanded upon and refined Weber's theory of social closure in a direction that enables us to take account of the strategies of occupations such as nursing. The first pertinent point that Parkin makes is that Weber placed too much emphasis on the arbitrary nature of the criteria that groups adopt to justify their social closure. In doing so, Weber failed to place enough emphasis on the role of the state in the process of social closure, in that groups are dependent upon the state accepting their criteria as appropriate if they are fully to succeed in attaining social closure. This point fits well with Freidson's (1970) argument that the autonomy that is at the core of professional activity is a deliberately granted autonomy, one which enjoys legal sanction.

The second point of Parkin's that I wish to discuss is his identification of other strategies of social closure. Parkin characterises Weber's model as 'social closure as exclusion': 'By social closure Weber means the process by which social collectivities seek to maximize rewards by restricting access to resources and opportunities to a limited circle of eligibles' (Parkin 1979: 44). However, what of those groups that have been excluded by the successful application of social closure? Parkin argues that, in many cases, they are not satisfied to let matters rest. Instead of accepting the position of the group that has excluded them, excluded groups will often attempt to break into the privileged ranks in order to have their own bite at the cherry, adopting a process that Parkin terms 'social closure as usurpation':

> Usurpation is that type of social closure mounted by a group in response to its outsider status and the collective experiences of exclusion. What usurpationary actions have in common is the aim of biting into the resources and benefits accruing to dominant groups in society – a range of possibilities extending from marginal redistribution to complete expropriation.
>
> (Parkin 1979: 74)

From Parkin's model, we can see that social closure is a highly contested process. On the one hand, there are groups attempting to maintain closure because of the advantages they enjoy through their exclusion of competitors. On the other hand, there are groups attempting to challenge or usurp that social closure in order to gain advantages from which they are currently excluded. These might seem to be opposite and contradictory strategies. However, Parkin argues that they may, in certain circumstances, be combined. Thus a status group or class may simultaneously attempt to break the monopoly over privileges that those of higher social or economic rank enjoy (social closure as usurpation) while at the same time attempting to prevent those of a lower rank poaching their own privileges (social closure as exclusion). Thus, in his discussion of the strategies employed by organised workers, Parkin argues that they 'frequently resort to *dual* forms of closure: usurpationary activities against employers and the state, combined with exclusionary activities against other less organized groups of workers, including ethnic minorities and women' (1979: 91).

Writers such as Anne Witz (1992) have argued that the strategies of occupations such as nursing and midwifery can be characterised as entailing dual closure strategies, which involve attempts both to usurp medical power and to exclude others from midwifery and nursing through the tactic of professional registration. Witz's work forms part of a body of analysis focusing on the attempts of occupations who do not perceive themselves as having gained full professional status but who aspire to do so. It also involves a progression upon the work examined thus far, in that it brings to the foreground an aspect of professionalism that has not been addressed, namely that of the effects of gender upon occupational status and market position.

Gender and professions

While accepting many of the arguments put forward by neo-Weberian theorists about the nature of professions, feminist commentators have argued that it is important to address the issue of women's position within society. Thus, for example, Crompton notes that:

> Within the corpus of stratification theory neither Marxist not Weberian class categories are particularly helpful in this respect; both market-derived and labour exploitation theories are gender-blind.
>
> (1987: 424)

This gender blindness has led malestream analysts of professions to associate professions exclusively with maleness. One of the primary aims of feminist occupational analysis has been to break this association:

> It is necessary to map out a less androcentric [male-centred] terrain within which to locate discussions of professions and patriarchy. The generic concept of profession is also a gendered one. It takes what are in fact the successful professional projects of class-privileged, male actors at a particular point in history to be the paradigmatic case of profession. So the first step towards purging analyses of their androcentric bias is to abandon any generic concept of profession and redefine the sociology of professions as the sociological history of occupations as individual, empirical and above all historical cases rather than as specimens of a more general, fixed concept.
>
> (Witz 1992: 64)

It should be noted that Witz's emphasis on difference does not entail the abandonment of general explanatory models, in that she advocates the use of Weberian conceptual tools, modified to take account of the processes of gender exclusion, as being the most appropriate theoretical approach to the analysis of professions (Witz 1990). Perhaps the best way of illustrating how Witz believes this can be done is to examine her account of the campaign at the start of the twentieth century for nursing registration.

Nursing example: registration and dual closure

The campaign for nursing registration started in earnest in 1887 with the formation of the British Nurses Association (the epithet 'Royal' later being added). This body was formed as a breakaway body from the Hospitals' Association as a result of nurses' dissatisfaction with the Hospitals' Association's antipathy to the autonomous registration of nurses. The leader of the campaign for registration was the ex-Matron of St Bartholemew's Hospital, Mrs Bedford-Fenwick. The campaign was far from being an easy one, vociferous opposition coming from the voluntary hospitals, segments of the medical profession and indeed from within nursing itself, most notably in the figure of Florence Nightingale. Opposition within nursing was sufficiently strong for the anti-registrationists to take control of the Royal British Nurses Association, forcing the pro-registrationists to regroup in 1902 under the banner of the Society for the State Registration of Trained Nurses. Eventually, the Nurses Registration Act was passed in 1919. However, as we shall see, the contents of that Act fell far short of the aspirations of Bedford-Fenwick and the pro-registrationists.

The aim of the campaign was the incorporation of a central statutory body for nursing that would be under the control of nurses. It was planned that this body would control entry into the profession of nurses. It would have the power to decide the length and content of nurse training. Entry to the profession would be uniportal (that is, there would only be one route to becoming a registered nurse).

Social closure as exclusion

Witz (1992) argues that the campaign for nursing registration can be characterised as a dual closure strategy as it contained both exclusionary and usurpationary dimensions. In terms of exclusionary strategies, the nursing reformers' aim was to 'form nursing into a distinct profession [and] clearly define who are and who are not real members of the profession' (*Nursing Record* 1888: 26, quoted by Witz 1992: 133). They were quite clear that nursing should not be open to all women but rather be restricted to a privileged group of 'educated' and 'cultured' women. In other words, the registration movement aspired to social closure on a class basis, which involved the exclusion of working class women, who had provided the core of the occupation prior to the Nightingale reforms.

Witz identifies three exclusionary elements to the campaign. The first of these was the demand for a centralised system of control over the occupation. This system of control was to be independent of other areas of authority, such as hospital management boards. The aim was to persuade the state to sponsor the creation of a nursing council that would have the power both to regulate the supply of labour and to ensure that something approaching a monopoly of practice was instituted. Here, we can see evidence that the nursing reformers were adopting strategies involving the classical moves of established professions, as described by neo-Weberian commentators, namely the creation of monopoly and the minimisation of supply through acceptance by the state of their professional claims.

Even if a council had been set up with the powers that the pro-registration reformers desired, this would not automatically have meant that control would lie in the hands of nurses. In order to ensure that it did, the reformers included a second demand that nurses should have the right to govern themselves. In order to achieve occupational autonomy, it was proposed that a majority of the members of the nurses' controlling body should themselves be nurses and that they should be directly elected by registered nurses. Bedford-Fenwick was very clear on the importance of this demand, arguing that if proposals that did not provide for self-government were passed, control would lie with a 'combined oligarchy of medical and lay employers' who would act to betray the interests of nursing and to deprive nurses of all responsibility in order to maintain their own professional power (quoted by Witz 1992: 149).

The third exclusionary strategy involved the demand of a uniportal system of entry into the occupation. The importance of there being only one route of entry was that it allowed for centralised control over the training curriculum, as well as over the length and standard of nurse education. Once again, we come back to the Weberian identification of 'specialist examinations' as tactical ploys used to facilitate the 'desire to limit the supply of candidates for... positions and to monopolize them for the holders of educational patents' (Weber 1968b: 1000).

Social closure as usurpation

It might seem from the above account that the registration campaign was largely about keeping undesirables out, limiting the supply of nurses and providing the profession with a monopoly over nursing practice – all of which looks little different from the strategies adopted by the 'male' professions. However, as Witz observes, the campaign also entailed a strong challenge to existing social arrangements, challenging the power of at least three sets of social élites.

The first élite challenged by the pro-registrationist movement was the managers of voluntary hospitals. These privately funded institutions had, under the Nightingale system of training, provided the seed-bed in which nurse training schools developed. These hospitals had benefited greatly from the Nightingale system, in that it had provided a cheap and compliant workforce. At the time of the registration movement, three-quarters of the nurses employed by hospitals were trainees, whose employment costs consisted only of the price of a room in which to live and a nominal wage (Maggs 1983).

During this era, the voluntary hospitals were enjoying a period of considerable growth. This meant that their demand for nursing labour was extremely high. Here we come back to the Weberian emphasis on the importance of market supply and demand. In terms of demand, the voluntary hospitals required an ever-larger number of nurses to fill the posts that resulted from their expansion. In accordance with the laws of the market, unless there was also a high level of supply, the prices that nurses could charge for their services would rise in response to the scarcity of their skills. In order to obviate this rise in price, which would have compromised their own profit margins, the voluntary hospitals wished to maintain a supply of cheap labour. State registration, by restricting both the number of trained nurses to those whom the regulatory body saw fit to admit, and also by restricting trainees to those who had attained the requisite qualifications for entry into training, would have the effect of severely restricting the supply of nurses. According to market laws, this restriction of supply would have the effect of raising market price. Thus, for many hospital managers, registered nurses simply meant expensive nurses.

The challenge that the reformers posed for hospital managers was not just an economic one: there was also the issue of control. Both registration and control over training threatened the power that the voluntary hospitals currently had over nurses:

> If the hospitals allowed the occupation to organize itself and create a more homogenous market, they recognized that their influence would be matched by that of a monopolistic supplier of nursing labour. Instead of nurses working on terms set by the hospitals, the hospitals would have to employ nurses on terms set by the occupation.
>
> (Dingwall *et al*. 1988: 81)

To summarise, in terms of both market position and occupational autonomy, the registration movement threatened to usurp the considerable powers that the voluntary hospital authorities enjoyed over their workforce.

As well as challenging the power of the hospital authorities, registration also threatened to alter the power relations that existed between doctors and nurses. However, as Witz notes, it is easy to overstate the challenge that the registrationists were posing to physicians. Indeed, by contemporary standards, the aspirations of the registrationists will seem almost timid. They had no thought of usurping medical control over nursing practice. Bedford-Fenwick was quite clear on this point, going so far as to state that part of the purpose of registration was 'to ensure that members of the Nursing Profession of the future should remain under the supervision of medical men' (*Nursing Record* 1888: 249, quoted by Witz 1992: 153). The aim of registration was not to give nurses discretion over the practical activities of nursing. Instead, the challenge to medicine came in the form of the assertion that nurses should have autonomy over the way in which their occupation was organised. While nurses still had a duty to obey physicians' practical orders, that did not extend to medicine having a right to control the occupational infrastructure of nursing.

Given these rather modest demands for autonomy from medicine, it is not surprising that the response of physicians to the registrationists' demands was ambiguous. Some groups within the medical profession opposed registration. Notable here were GPs, who feared that registration would encourage clients to consult nurses for many of the ailments that they would previously have taken to physicians, thus challenging the monopoly that GPs currently enjoyed. However, many physicians were highly supportive. Indeed, in 1895, the British Medical Association resolved to support nurse registration, although at the price of medical representation on the nursing council.

The third set of power relations that was challenged by the campaign for registration was that of gendered relations. The pro-registrationists were quite clear that their demands for self-government were based on the rights of women to work independently of male control, in this case in the form of male administrators and physicians:

> The relation between nursing and medicine was articulated as a gendered relation. It was not simply the case that nurses as an occupational group strove for a measure of independence from medicine, but it was also the case that they articulated their common interests as women in the medical division of labour.
>
> (Witz 1992: 154)

It will be remembered that the registration campaign was going on at the same time as the campaign for women's suffrage. Indeed, it might be viewed as another arm of the of the early feminist movement, the suffragettes articulating the demand for women's right to a more equal position within the polity and the pro-registrationists demanding more equality in the workplace. It is in the construction of registration as a women's issue that the gendered nature of nursing's dual closure strategy is most clearly demonstrated. Registration was not simply a matter of inter-occupational jockeying, but was also an attempt significantly move to the boundaries of the gendered power relations that working women experienced.

The failure and success of registration

While registration was eventually granted by Parliament in 1919, the form that it took fell far short of the demands of the pro-registrationists. True, a centralised body with a majority of nursing representatives was set up, in the form of the General Nursing Council. However, the powers of that body were extremely limited. It had no control over the pay and conditions of nurses, or over the content of nursing examinations, and the aspiration of uniportal entry was denied. Moreover, the Council did not have the autonomy to make rules on its own: these had to be put before Parliament before they could be enacted. Thus, the tactic of using educational credentials and professional monopoly, which, in promising to improve the market and status position of nursing, threatened the position of powerful élites, was thwarted. In Witz's words, the outcome of the registration campaign represented a failure of this female professional project.

However, as we all know, the story did not end there. While it may have taken over 60 years to get things moving, the aims of this female professional project were, by the 1980s, once again being advanced. With the setting up of the United Kingdom Central Council for Nursing, Midwifery and Health Visiting, constituted by a majority of members elected by practitioners, and having the power to set and police professional rules, to control registration and to institute a uniportal system of entry in the form of the Project 2000 reforms, the strategy of social closure appeared to be succeeding. These developments have since been reinforced by the mass migration of nurse training into the higher education sector, which has considerably raised the status value of 'specialist examinations'. Approaching contemporary nursing from this perspective, it looks as if things are going very well. However, progress may be less rapid than it would appear.

Nursing example: the limits of social closure

In a paper entitled 'Northern nursing: the limits of idealism' (Porter 1995b), I examined the degree to which the occupational strategies of nursing have succeeded in altering the position of clinical nurses, especially in relation to their medical colleagues. One of the strategies I addressed was that of the nursing process. I argued that the development of the nursing process is a prime example of a dual closure strategy. On the one hand, it is usurpationary, in that it challenges the previous medical monopoly over diagnosis and prescription. Thus, the 1983 Statutory Instruments of the Nurses, Midwives and Health Visitors Act provided state sanction for nursing diagnosis and prescription as a formal remit of appropriately qualified nurses. At the same time, it is exclusionary, in that those Statutory Instruments also specified that it was only first-level nurses who were to be allowed to devise and assess nursing process care plans, thus excluding those nurses who did not possess the requisite professional registration. Specifically, the second-class status of enrolled nurses was copperfastened.

In order to see how the nursing process affected the working lives of nurses, I chose the case study of an intensive care unit in which the nursing process was being operated through the medium of the Roper, Logan and Tierney (1985) model of nursing. Examination of the use of the process by nursing staff suggested an interesting paradox. While the nurses spent a great deal of effort going through the motions of filling in process documentation, they actually made very little use of the information they had gathered.

With the admission of each new patient, considerable time was spent filling in biographical details, assessing problems concerning the 12 activities of living, prescribing appropriate nursing actions and setting proposed outcomes for those actions, all in long hand. Apart from taking some personal details from relatives, most of documentation was completed by the nurse in isolation.

After initial formulation, the process documentation was revised three times daily, once again demanding considerable nursing time. When the time was not available, nurses prioritised the information they put into the process documentation. Information about the patient's condition and the effects of care were always written up contemporaneously, while information concerning the changing nature of the framework of care was often left until slack periods. Often time was not found until the weekend, when the nurses worked back over the documentation to reconstruct the progress of the previous week's care. It appeared that the nurses placed far more emphasis on the basic facts of care than they did on the nursing theory aspects of the plans; diagnosis, planning and evaluation were neglected in favour of data collection and the recording of treatment.

In practical terms, the nurses did not use the nursing process to facilitate communication, either with patients and relatives or between themselves. Between the three compulsory updates in the day, care plans were stored away and ignored. They were not even referred to during shift handovers. Instead, nurses relied on their memories and the observation charts in order to report to the oncoming nurse. Thus the first problem with the nursing process was its irrelevance to nursing care.

The second problem (in terms of the process' function as part of a dual closure strategy) was the content of care plans. Rather than demonstrating nursing autonomy, the way in which care plans were constructed tended to indicate a continuing medical dominance. This was a reflection of the fact that, despite nursing's formal remit to diagnose and prescribe in relation to nursing problems, many decisions about changes in the care regime could only be made by doctors. For example, nurses were not able to decide whether or when a patient required an intravenous infusion. Therefore, the planning of nursing care in relation to the activity of 'eating and drinking' was entirely dependent upon medical decisions about the appropriate medium of fluid intake. This is not to say that nurses were completely subservient to physicians: they had considerable informal input into decisions (see Porter 1991). However, notwithstanding this, it remained the case that most important decisions about care were made by physicians, nursing care plans being constructed in response to those decisions.

In the case of this intensive care unit, the formal attempt to improve the occupational status of nursing through the development of a diagnostic and prescriptive role failed because of a combination of medical power and nursing antipathy. Nurses realised that, for all the work they put into it, the process did not deliver the autonomy it promised. Indeed, the main reason that nurses bothered with care plans at all was to 'cover their asses' (to use J.M. Johnson's, 1972, quaint phrase). They realised that, even if they were not aids to care, care plans were legal documents that could be called upon in cases of litigation or disciplinary action. They also realised that gaps in these records would be likely to be interpreted as gaps in actual care. This is why nurses were so punctilious about filling in the 'facts' of the patient's condition and their care, and not so worried about other, more theoretical, aspects of the care plans.

It needs to be asked why the efforts of nursing reformers have not been entirely successful in achieving a greater degree of social closure. Probably the first thing to note is that the setting of the case study had a considerable effect, in that the highly technological nature of intensive care units may tend to promote medical dominance, whereas less technological settings, where the emphasis is more exclusively on care, could well favour a greater degree of nursing autonomy. However, even accepting this qualification, there remains a problem for those who wish to see dual closure aspirations having a practical effect upon the occupational position of clinical nurses.

One reason may be that nursing suffers from an excessive idealism, in the sense that there has been a tendency to put too much faith in good ideas without fully considering how material circumstances might promote or constrain the implementation of those ideas. In the case of the nursing process, it could be argued that nurses have attempted to use the process in order to copy the diagnostic autonomy that they see doctors enjoying, in the hope that this development within nursing will deliver something like the autonomy that medicine has gained from its monopolisation of diagnosis and prescription. However, what this fails to take into account is the significance of nursing's *relationship* with other occupational groups, namely medicine. In other words, while diagnostic autonomy may well be an essential prerequisite for occupational autonomy, that autonomy cannot simply be gained by the internal restructuring of nursing. What is also needed is for nurses to challenge the power relations that pertain between themselves and physicians, and, more fundamentally, the general social structures that generate those power relations.

The Marxist riposte

In a way, this theoretical explanation of the problems that some nurses have encountered in operationalising the nursing process (an explanation with which you may or may not agree) entails a quasi-Marxist critique of the dual closure strategy and its Weberian interpretation, in so far as it argues that, in order to understand occupational power relations, we need to look below the surface of the occupational market place and examine those forces which structure the market and the position of the various competing groups within it.

Marxists criticise the Weberian focus on market arrangements on the grounds that it is unable to explain why those market arrangements take the form they do, beyond pointing to the meaning systems that those involved in the market adopt (for example, identification of the connection between industrial society and the adoption of rational modes of thought). In contrast, Marxists argue that we need to look at the material conditions that pertain, irrespective of the subjective states of actors. The distinctiveness of capitalist societies lies in the form of exploitation that they entail, which is embedded in the relations of production between the owners and non-owners of the means of production. Indeed, it is in Marxism's concentration on exploitation, in contrast to Weberians' emphasis on market exchanges, that the core difference in their approaches to social inequality lies. Ironically, despite Weber's identification of a plurality of groups competing in the market place, Marxists argue that the effect of his analysis is to reduce all those groups to a common denominator of market competitor:

> The difference between viewing production from the vantage point of exchange or exploitation has significant implications for the kind of class theory that is built upon this foundation. For Weber, owners of capital, raw labour power and skills all meet in the market and are all part of a single class system or class logic because the exchanges take place within the institutional context. Marx, on the other hand, regards the distinctively capitalist class structure as only involving the exchange between capital and labour power because it is this exchange that generates the distinctively capitalist form of exploitation. Skill ownership is irrelevant to the specification of *capitalist* class relations.
>
> (Wright 1985: 107)

Perhaps this is to put the argument against the importance of skills and services too strongly. Even Wright himself (1989) has since come to accept that the relationship between the ownership and non-ownership of skills is one of the fundamental schisms in advanced industrial societies. Nevertheless, Marxists would still argue that it is important to understand why the market for skills and services takes the form it does, and as a consequence assert the need to address the fundamental structures of inequality and exploitation that shape that market.

These concluding critical remarks are unfortunately rather difficult and esoteric. However, they reflect one of the enduring debates within social theory: is the social world an objective reality that exists outside the meanings people construct of it, which as we have seen from Chapter 2, Durkheim believed; or is it the other way round, the social world being a construction of the interpretations that people have about what is going on around them? The next section of the book will turn to those theorists who adopt the latter interpretation, namely symbolic interactionists, social phenomenologists and ethnomethodologists.

Recommended further reading

For Weber's theory of class status and party, one can refer to Weber's own short piece on the issue in the volume edited by Gerth and Mills, entitled *From Max Weber* (Weber 1970). The most succinct secondary discussion is to be found in Chapter 4 of Frank Parkin's textbook, *Max Weber* (1982). A good recent text on the sociology of professions is provided by Keith MacDonald (1995). In addition, Anne Witz's *Professions and Patriarchy* (1992) provides an excellent review of both Marxist and Weberian perspectives on professions from a feminist standpoint. For a short critical analysis of nursing's professional project, see Porter's 'The poverty of professionalization' (1992). Further discussion of power and professionalism as they pertain to nursing can be found in Geoff Wilkinson's forthcoming volume in this series on power in nursing practice.

PART II

Getting to the action

This part will examine three theoretical positions that all operate under the common assumption that, if we wish to understand the social world, there is no point in looking to social structures. Social structures, if they exist at all, are merely the products of individual ideas and actions. As a result, examination of the social world should start with a study of individuals, how they interpret the world and how they interact with others on the basis of their interpretations.

There are numerous names for these approaches, interpretative, hermeneutic and action theories being the three most common. I have chosen to use the latter here simply because it gave the snappiest title. However, it is as good as any. It refers to Weber's (1968a [1922]) famous assertion that social action should be the central subject matter of sociology. In other words, if we want to understand society, we need to understand why social actors act in the ways in which they do. All three perspectives dealt with in this part – symbolic interactionism in Chapter 5 and phenomenology and ethnomethodology in Chapter 6 – engage, to a greater or lesser degree, in this project.

Why does this particular strand of social theory merit a section to itself, when its opposite – structuralism – does not? The reason for this is that structuralism has had relatively little impact upon nursing discourse, whereas action theories have. This is not hard to understand, given that nursing practice normally involves one-to-one interaction with clients. Given the nature of nursing work, there is obvious merit in being aware of action theories. However, as I noted in Chapter 1, objections have been made to the concentration on them in nursing education, on the grounds that they fail to recognise the significance of social structures upon health and health care (Cooke 1993a, 1993b). Looking forward to Part III, I hope to show that there is no longer a need to make a choice between either action theory or structuralism, in that theories have been constructed to take due account of the insights of both.

5 Symbolic interactionism, labelling and stigma

Introduction

Symbolic interactionism, as its name suggests, concentrates on the dynamics of interaction between individuals rather than on examining large-scale social structures. Its aim is to explain social actions and interactions in terms of the meanings that those actions have for social actors. It is unique in terms of the theories presented in this book in that it is almost exclusively a home-grown North American product rather than an extension of European social theory. The pertinence of this observation is that it has been argued that symbolic interactionism reflects to a large degree the American cultural ideals of individualism and freedom, in contrast to the European emphasis on the constraints and enablements of social structures such as social class (Shaskolsky 1970).

This chapter begins with an account of the general philosophical origins of symbolic interactionism, as is found in the ideas of George Herbert Mead. It then goes on to discuss its application to sociology by Mead's pupil, Herbert Blumer. From here, the chapter focuses on a specific aspect of symbolic interactionism, namely labelling theory, which argues that people in society are labelled as deviant not according to their innate attributes but instead according to the symbolic interpretations of those supposed attributes that others construct. This is related to the field of health through the discussion of Thomas Scheff's application of labelling theory to the area of mental illness. Staying on the theme of mental illness, Erving Goffman's critique of the degrading interactive processes of 'total institutions' is examined. Goffman's work on stigma is also addressed. Finally, an example of the use of symbolic interactionism to interrogate nursing practice is found in Alistair Hewison's paper 'Nurses' power in interactions with patients'.

George Herbert Mead's social psychology

While he did not use the actual term 'symbolic interactionism', George Herbert Mead (1863–1931) is commonly accepted as being the founder of this particular theoretical position. Mead published little during his lifetime, his influence coming initially through his lectures. Indeed, his most important book was the posthumously published collection of lectures notes entitled *Mind, Self and Society* (Mead 1934). Mead's concerns were essentially philosophical: his focus of enquiry was the nature of the human self.

The first thing that we need to address is what he meant by the 'self'. According to Mead, we only have a self if we can regard ourselves as objects – if we can examine and evaluate our own thought processes in much the same way that we would examine and evaluate other things and ideas that we come across. Having a self involves the ability to reflect upon one's mental processes. It is the capacity to engage in this 'inner conversation' that enables our actions to be something more than automatic responses to stimuli, because it enables us to think about our responses. This capacity to think back on one's thoughts and activities is termed 'reflexivity': It is, according to Mead, what distinguishes humans from other animals.

The next obvious question concerns how one gains the ability to treat one's mind as an object – to see oneself as others see one. The key to this capacity, according to Mead, is the childhood process of socialisation. Mead argues that there are two stages to the development of the self. In the first stage, children play at being other individuals, such as their mother or father. However, once they begin to play games that involve a number of individuals, they develop an awareness of their relationship with other players and begin to gain an understanding of the collective viewpoint of others around them. In Mead's words, they take on the attitude of the 'generalised other'.

Mead's close collaborator, Charles Horton Cooley (1864–1929), put this argument even more starkly. He argued that the connection between society and the individual self was inextricable, that 'self and society are twin-born' (1942: 5). For Cooley, there could be no such thing as an isolated self. The self only develops through our incorporation of the views of others; it is, in his memorable phrase, a 'looking-glass self'. This relationship between social groups and the individual assumes certain qualities on the part of the individual, most importantly the capacity to apprehend, interpret and incorporate the views of those with whom we come into contact, in short the ability to engage in symbolic interaction.

An act only becomes symbolic if there is a shared meaning attached to it. Thus, the significance of the shapes on this page is that they are symbolic of concepts, and that awareness of the relationship between the symbol and what it represents is shared by all those with access to the linguistic culture of English. The common symbolism of the English language (I hope) enables me as a writer to share meanings with you, the reader. Thus, you and I are, albeit at a distance, engaging in symbolic communication.

A symbol does not simply stand for something that is already there. According to Mead, the meaning that we attach to an object is the result not of the innate qualities of that object but of the active interpretation that we put upon it. Take, for example, an accident and emergency department. The cultural significance of such a department lies in people's expectation that if, having interpreted themselves as being sick or injured, they go to one, they will be seen by a professional health care worker who will assess what is wrong with them and decide what is best to be done. There is nothing in the physical reality of an accident and emergency department that requires any of these activities. It could be used as an office, a living area or a school. Its relevance to the lives of those who use it lies in the way it has been symbolically constructed. This is a social matter: it involves a shared cultural heritage that contains assumptions about appropriate forms of health care. Thus, the symbols we use to interpret the world around us are inherently social.

Herbert Blumer's definition

It was one of Mead's students at the University of Chicago, Herbert Blumer, who actually coined the term 'symbolic interactionism', which he saw as referring:

> to the peculiar and distinctive character of interaction as it takes place between human beings. The peculiarity consists in the fact that human

beings interpret or 'define' each other's actions instead of merely reacting to each other's actions. Their 'response' is not made directly to the actions of one another but instead is based on the meaning which they attach to such actions. Thus, human interaction is mediated by the use of symbols, by interpretation, or by ascertaining the meaning of one another's actions.

(Blumer 1962: 180)

It was Blumer who explicitly developed symbolic interactionism as a social theory rather than a philosophical position. His achievement was to draw out the implicitly sociological in Mead's work and render it explicit.

Blumer argued that symbolic interactionism rested on three basic premises. The first premise was that 'human beings act towards things on the basis of the meanings that the things have for them' (1969: 2). By 'things', he meant everything that humans might come across: physical objects, other human beings, institutions, ideals, activities and situations. This first premise may seem to be a fairly uncontentious assumption, in that all it is saying is that we use our minds when we act – we interpret what is going on around us and act on the basis of the interpretation that we make. However, Blumer argued that while such a position might seem obvious, many scholars had forgotten it. The historical context of Blumer's work is important here. At the time he was writing, there was a tendency in both social and psychological theorists to see people's behaviour as being determined by outside factors. Thus, psychological behaviourists such as Watson and Skinner concentrated on stimulus response and tended to dismiss the importance of consciousness. At the other end of the spectrum, were, as we shall see, those sociologists who tended to regard human behaviour as a response to the influences of social structures. Blumer rejected both of these positions, arguing that rather than being passive recipients of external determining factors, human beings are active organisms in their own right. To understand behaviour, it is insufficient simply to identify the factors that influence that behaviour. Because the meanings that things have for people are crucial in their own right, an adequate explanation of behaviour must take account of them.

The second premise of symbolic interactionism involved a rejection of the idea that meaning came from the intrinsic qualities of things or that it was generated by the internal psychology of people. Instead, Blumer argued that meaning arises from the process of interaction between people:

> The meaning of a thing for a person grows out of the ways in which other persons act toward the person with regard to the thing. Their actions operate to define the thing for the person. Thus, symbolic interactionism sees meanings as social products, as creations that are formed in and through defining activities of people as they interact.
>
> (1969: 4–5)

Here, we can clearly see the sociological aspect of symbolic interactionism: because the meanings upon which we base our actions are social products, our social environment is central to our very humanity. However, Blumer sees a danger in putting this argument forward too strongly, in that it brings us back to the idea that humans are passive recipients of external determining factors, that the meanings that we have simply involve the automatic application of already established meanings that come to us through our interaction with others.

The third premise, that 'meanings are handled in, and modified through, an interpretative process used by the person in dealing with the things he encounters' (1969: 2), involves a rejection of the social determination of meanings. Blumer argues that this 'interpretative process' involves what might be termed an internal conversation: it entails the person interacting with herself. This returns us to Mead's idea of selfhood being the capacity to reflect upon one's own mental processes. On the basis of this communication, the person is able to select, modify, check or reject socially generated meanings in the light of her situation and aims. Thus, there is nothing automatic about our use of meanings – rather than accepting them wholesale, we revise and adapt them. In short, rather than determining our actions, Blumer argues that socially generated meanings can be better seen as instruments for the guidance of human action.

Because human interaction is an ongoing process involving participants developing lines of conduct on the basis of their interpretation of their situation, Blumer argues that the established patterns of social life (in other words, social structures) do not exist independently of those interpretations. If the meanings, definitions and interpretations that sustain an established pattern of social life are undermined, the pattern itself will collapse. In short, the essence of society lies in the interactions of its members. Therefore, to be understood, society must be analysed in terms of the actions that sustain it. This has important consequences for the approach that the researcher is required to adopt. Rather than taking a detached, 'objective' approach, viewing social actions from the outside, it is incumbent upon the researcher to see the social world from the standpoint of the actor, in order to see how she perceives and attaches meaning to her social world and organises her actions accordingly (Blumer 1966).

Labelling theory

Having laid out the general theoretical foundations of symbolic interactionism as formulated by Mead and Blumer, I now wish to discuss two more specific approaches to the social world that rely heavily on this theoretical standpoint. These are labelling theory and the work of Erving Goffman.

Howard Becker built his labelling theory of deviance up from two basic symbolic interactionist premises: first, that our self is the result of neither biological nor social structural imperatives but rather of the symbolic interpretations that emerge from our inter-action with others; second, that the meaning that we attach to an object is the result not of the innate qualities of that object but of the active interpretation that we put upon it. Accordingly, he regarded deviance from social norms not as a given fact but as a result of the interpretations that members of society apply to certain individuals. He stated:

> deviance is *not* a quality of the act the person commits, but rather a consequence of the application by others of rules and sanctions to an 'offender'. The deviant is one to whom that label has been successfully applied; deviant behavior is behavior that people so label.
>
> (Becker 1963: 9)

By saying this, Becker was not trying to imply that people labelled as deviant had not committed the act that they were accused of committing. However, he was arguing that we could not assume that this was the case. Because the process of labelling is not infallible, people might be labelled without having broken the social rule that they have been accused of breaking. Similarly, people may break rules and get away with it, avoiding the label being applied to them. Taking this sort of line, the interesting question no longer concerns the factors that can account for a supposed act of deviance. Rather, such an analysis concentrates on:

> deviance as the product of a transaction that takes place between some social group and one who is viewed by the group as a rule-breaker.
>
> (Becker 1963: 10)

Basically, Becker's position is that whether an act is deviant or not depends on how other people react to it.

Mental illness as labelled deviance

Labelling theory has been applied by Thomas Scheff to the explanation of mental illness. Scheff regards psychiatric symptoms not so much as results of internal psychological dysfunction but as 'labelled violations of social norms' (Scheff 1966: 25). He calls the type of social norms involved 'residual rules'. These are the social conventions that are considered so 'natural' that they are not governed by explicit rules. To illustrate his point, Scheff takes an example from Goffman's book *Behavior in Public Places* (1964). Goffman notes that there is a general social norm of 'involvement' in public places or, put another way, a rule against 'having no purpose'. This leads to strategies that provide a respectable veneer to lolling about doing nothing. Instead of sitting by a river bank, people fish; instead of sleeping on a beach, they 'get a tan'. Now, there is no explicit social rule that says 'Thou shalt not lie around doing absolutely nothing'; however, such a requirement is an implicit, taken-for-granted social norm. Those who loll about in public without an acceptable pretext for doing so are therefore seen as violating a residual rule.

Scheff argues that we all, at some time or another, break residual rules. However, not all of us are labelled as mentally ill. What then leads some residual rule-breakers to be labelled as deviant? Scheff's answer is that the most important single factor lies not in the behaviour of the rule-breaker but in societal reaction. This involves the application of the stereotype of mental illness. Whether or not this stereotype is applied depends on a number of factors, including the amount of tolerance that the community has for the act committed, the status and power of the rule-breaker and the availability of alternative, more innocuous explanations. Once labelled as mentally ill, Scheff argues that the person has been launched on a deviant 'career'. Those who are labelled will usually be rewarded for adopting the stereotypical role of mental illness, while if they attempt to resist it and assert their normality, they will tend to be punished. It might be argued that here Scheff is contradicting Blumer's third premise that meanings are interpreted and modified by the individual, that they do not accept social meanings without question. However, Scheff points out that in the personal 'crisis that is occurring when a residual rule-breaker is being publicly labelled, the deviant is highly suggestible, and may accept the proffered role of the insane as the only alternative' (1966: 88).

This application of labelling theory has not been accepted by all sociologists. Most notably, Walter Gove (1980) has argued that Scheff is simply incorrect in his description of the career of the mental patient. He argues that mental illness cannot simply be seen as residual rule-breaking, in that the majority of people so labelled quite evidently have a serious disorder. Moreover, rather than being coerced into adopting the stereotype of mental illness, many people are screened out by mental health professionals, and many others, following treatment, are able to put their experience behind them, without becoming institutionalised.

Total institutions

The idea of the experience of mental illness as a career has also been applied by Erving Goffman in *Asylums* (1968a [1961]). Like Scheff, Goffman uses the term 'career' not in the sense of occupational development but rather in the more general sense of referring to any social strand of a person's course through life. In addressing what he terms 'the moral career of the mental patient', Goffman is concentrating upon 'the regular sequence of changes that career entails in the person's self and in his framework of imagery for judging himself and others' (1968a: 119). Goffman identifies three major stages in this moral career – pre-patient, in-patient and ex-patient. Concentrating on the first two stages, Goffman graphically demonstrates the 'mortification of the self' – the stripping away of a person's original identity – that is involved. In the pre-patient stage, the typical scenario is one in which significant others come to the decision that psychiatric care is appropriate. This has significant ramifications for the pre-patient's interpersonal relationships and sense of self:

> he starts out with relationships and rights, and ends up, at the beginning of his hospital stay, with hardly any of either. The moral aspects of this career, then, typically begin with the experience of abandonment, disloyalty and embitterment.
>
> (Goffman 1968a: 125)

The cruellest blow to bear is what the pre-patient often sees as the betrayal of those closest to them. They discover that those to whom they turn for help in response to the threat of incarceration are themselves implicated in the process, often collaborating with psychiatric professionals. Thus, the most familiar social props of the pre-patient's world are stripped away, to the point at which the pre-patient may finally come to the conclusion 'that he has been deserted by society and turned out of relationships by those closest to him' (1968a: 135).

This process of the mortification of the self continues with a vengeance during the in-patient stage. At this point, the person enters what Goffman terms a 'total institution', an institution cut off from the rest of the social world, where inmates sleep, play and work in the same place, where they live communally with a large number of fellow inmates who are all treated alike, and where daily activities are tightly scheduled by formal rules that are applied by a body of officials. One of the consequences of entering such an institution is that the normal props of personality, such as freedom of movement, personalised clothing and privacy, are denied. The patient begins to learn how difficult it is to maintain a conception of oneself as a human individual when the usual social supports for that conception are removed. Moreover, it is impressed upon the in-patient that she has failed in her life and therefore no longer deserves the status normally accorded adult members of society. In reaction to this, the patient may attempt to construct a personal history that minimises her responsibility for what has occurred to her. In other words, she will attempt to construct a story of her life that will minimise the sense of shame that she is experiencing. However, this attempt at the reconstruction of a respectable self comes into conflict with the interests of professional staff, who wish to see the patient accept her difficulties and thus co-operate with the psychiatric treatments that have been prescribed to cure those difficulties. Staff, therefore, have much to gain from breaking down this last line of defence that the patient has erected in order to maintain a creditable self. They do this by challenging claims that involve the denial of respon-sibility and by emphasising those aspects of a person's history that are most discrediting:

> In general, then, mental hospitals systematically provide for circulation about each patient the kind of information that the patient is likely to try to hide. And in various degrees of detail this information is used daily to puncture his claims. At the admission and diagnostic conferences, he will be asked questions to which he must give wrong answers in order to maintain his self-respect, and then the true answer will be shot back at him.
>
> (1968a: 148–9)

This process may be repeated through numerous cycles, and each time it occurs, the patient's sense of what a person ought to be forces her to reconstruct her story; each time she does so, staff may respond by discrediting her story once again.

Where does all this lead the person whose self has been so mortified? Goffman suggests two career trajectories. One possi-bility is the rebirth of the self as model patient. In this scenario, the professional psychiatric outlook is fully accepted. The other possi-bility is one in which, in Goffman's words, the patient learns to practise 'the amoral arts of shamelessness' (1968a: 155). Here, the patient comes to accept that she can survive without what is socially construed as a viable self and therefore ceases serious attempts at defending the self against the efforts of psychiatric staff to debunk it. From this perspective of apathy, the process of building up a self just to have it destroyed simply becomes a shameless game.

What are we to make of this rather dark application of symbolic interactionism to the world of psychiatric care? One thing to note is that it was written 35 years ago, and things have changed considerably since then. Indeed, the impact of *Asylums* contributed in no small way to people's attitudes towards psychiatric institutions and thus gave momentum to the move towards community care, which, it might be argued, has altered the dynamics of professional/client interaction.

At a more theoretical level, it might be noted that the path of the moral career, as traced by Goffman, is altogether too straight and narrow to be accommodated within the tenets of symbolic interactionism. While it adheres closely to Blumer's second premise that our interpretations of life arise out of social interaction with those around us, it does not fit so well with the third premise that socially generated meanings, rather than determining our actions, can be better seen as instruments for our guidance. While Goffman does present us with different possible responses to the process of mortification, it has become received wisdom in the literature that this process is an inevitable consequence of being admitted to a total institution. This view has recently been challenged by Pauline Prior (1995), who has used a case study analysis of a psychiatric hospital in-patient of 36 years standing to challenge the notion of the all-pervading power of the total institution. On the basis of this patient's capacity to maintain his personal identity throughout the period of his incarceration, she argues that it is possible to survive long-term institutional psychiatric care without being completely resocialised. She notes that one of the factors affecting survival chances is the strength of an individual's personal identity. This exception to the rule, as it were, reminds us of the symbolic interactionist assertion that, to understand behaviour, it is insufficient simply to identify the factors that influence that behaviour, in that we also have to look at the meanings that people apply to those factors.

Stigma

Goffman's contribution to the connection between social theory and health and health care knowledge is not limited to his work on asylums. He also penned an extremely influential book dealing with the issue of social stigma. In *Stigma* (1968b [1963]), Goffman examines the effects upon an individual that result from the application to her of a stigmatising label.

His work on stigma was the specific application of his more general theory about people's roles in social interaction. Following Cooley's notion of the looking-glass self, Goffman believed not only that our sense of ourselves is closely bound up with how others see us, but also that we realise that this is so. Thus, in order to foster a sense of self-esteem, we will make an effort to present ourselves to others as worthy of esteem. To do this, we will engage in what Goffman terms 'impression management' (1969 [1959]). This involves performing in such a way as to control the impression that others have of us that will lead them to see us as commendable. Goffman's view of how people act towards each other is very much like play-acting. He sees us as projecting not some sort of inner, essential self that is really us but a series of roles or parts, which will change depending upon our audience. For example, the nurse whom the patient sees while the nurse is 'front stage' may be a rather different person from the nurse whom her colleagues see 'back stage'. Front stage, the nurse will be politely formal and professionally discreet, never thinking of uttering an expletive, despite the fact that she is being bossed about by a junior house officer, barely out of college, while she is trying to perform a procedure. However, back stage in the coffee room, her approach may well be considerably more abrasive. Thus, for Goffman, life is just a series of dramatic performances. Reflecting this, he describes his theoretical perspective as the dramaturgical approach.

For most of us for most of the time, our impression management works, and we are accorded to a greater or lesser degree the respect that we seek to foster. However, for many people, the drama of impression management is considerably more problematic. These are people who have been stigmatised. Before going any further, we should be clear about what Goffman means by the term 'stigma'.

Goffman argues that every society has stereotypical expectations about how individuals ought to be. Goffman terms these expectations, which we bring to bear in our routine social interactions with others, 'virtual social identity'. However, some people's 'actual social identity' – the attributes that they actually possess – does not match these stereotypes. It is this discrepancy between virtual social identity and actual social identity, between social expectations and individual reality, that generates stigma. It should be noted that this is not simply a matter of difference; it also implies a moral judgement in that stigma is a difference that is deeply discrediting. Indeed, Goffman goes so far to argue that we do not see people with stigmas as fully human. This image of the stigmatised as being inferior to 'normals' results in all sorts of discrimination, and in rationalisations for that discrimination. Nor is it just 'normals' who accept this moral evaluation. The influence of the interpretations of the wider society upon the stigmatised causes them to perceive their own attributes as being defiling things to possess. Thus, Goffman contends that 'shame becomes a central possibility' in the lives of the stigmatised (1968b: 18).

It is important to note that stigma cannot be read off from the nature of a specific attribute. We recall the symbolic interactionist rejection of the idea that meaning results from the intrinsic quality of things in favour of the assertion that meanings are social products. Thus, for example, many people would find the need to avail of psychiatric care, with the attendant label of being mentally ill, a very stigmatising experience. However, if one is a well-heeled New Yorker, attending a psychoanalyst is (if we are to believe Woody Allen) almost a status symbol.

Goffman describes how stigma deeply affects the social worlds of those who have been stigmatised. Social interaction with 'normals' is fraught with difficulties. One of these is that the stigma will be in the forefront of both their minds. Not only does this make the stigmatised feel very self-conscious, but it can also lead the 'normal' person to distort her interpretation of what should be everyday events. Thus, a minor accomplishment on the part of the stigmatised may be regarded as a sign of a remarkable capacity, while a minor failing may be interpreted as a direct result of the person's stigmatised difference. Despite these exaggerated responses, it is likely that the normal will pretend not even to notice the discredited attribute of the stigmatised. This very self-conscious 'disattention' adds to the difficulties of interaction in that 'the situation can become tense, uncertain, and ambiguous for all participants, especially the stigmatized one' (Goffman 1968b: 57). In short, impression management of a 'spoiled identity' is a very difficult task indeed. It is not surprising that the very anticipation of such contacts can lead the stigmatised to avoid them, leading to problems such as depression and anxiety that result from social isolation.

However, not everyone presents such interactional problems for the stigmatised. Goffman identifies two groups in which the stigmatised will be seen as fully human rather than discredited. These he terms the 'own' and the 'wise'. The own are those who have a similar stigma applied to them and who can therefore empathise on the basis of their own experiences. The wise are those who are 'normal' but whose particular situation gives them access to, and sympathy for, the secret life of the stigmatised individual and who come to accept her for what she is. One type of wise person is the one whose wisdom comes from working in an occupation that caters for the wants of the stigmatised. It is into this category that nurses may fit. Of course, the development from familiarity to acceptance is not an automatic process. The 'normal' nurse must first of all come to see the stigmatised other as an ordinary individual. Second, this interpretation must be accepted by the stigmatised.

Not all attributes open to social stigma are immediately apparent. Goffman makes the distinction between the 'discredited' – where the attribute that differs from stereotypical expectations is evident – and the 'discreditable', in which a person's 'differentness' is not immediately apparent. For the latter group, impression management entails different strategies:

> The issue is not that of managing tension generated during social contacts, but rather that of managing information about his failing. To display or not to display; to tell or not to tell; to lie or not to lie; and in each case, to whom, how, when, and where.
>
> (Goffman 1968b: 57)

In other words, the problem for the discreditable is to work out just how much information about themselves it is wise or safe to disclose to others. At least two strategies can be adopted here. The first Goffman calls 'passing', by which he means that the person will attempt to pass herself off as not having the attribute that is regarded as stigmatising. Here, we might think of the person who is hard of hearing who wears an unobtrusive hearing aid, or the person with diabetes who administers her insulin injections surreptitiously. Passing strategies will often be developed in collaboration with close others. Thus, the partner of a person with a colostomy may routinely check for odours before the person leaves the house.

However, there is always the danger of an embarrassing incident during which the stigma becomes publicly known despite the person's best efforts. For example, a person with epilepsy who suffers a public grand mal fit will pass dramatically and embarrassingly from discreditable to discredited. Some people, rather than constantly living in fear of exposure, prefer to manage the disclosure of information on their own terms.

The second strategy involves admission by the person that she has a stigma, along with a simultaneous effort to minimise the obtrusiveness of the stigma. An example given by Goffman relates to a blind person who is also facially disfigured. Such a person may choose to wear dark glasses in public. The glasses serve the dual purpose of indicating the person's blindness and also hiding the disfigurement.

From this discussion, it might seem that Goffman wants to divide the world into two camps: the 'normal' and the 'stigmatised'. However, he develops his argument in a rather disconcerting direction. For Goffman, we are all, to greater or lesser degrees, carriers of stigma: 'The most fortunate of normals is likely to have his half-hidden failing, and for every little failing there is a social occasion when it will loom large' (1968b: 127). We all, therefore, engage in the game of impression management and attempt to optimise our image as others see it.

We can see from Goffman's work on stigma that symbolic interactionist insights into the degree to which our individual selves are bound up with those around us leads to very distressing problems when those around us fail to afford us full recognition of our humanity. However, we need to ask whether his portrayal of social life as play-acting between individuals is an adequate one. For one thing, the idea of a structured society becomes difficult to sustain. As Alvin Gouldner (1971: 380) observes:

> Such social order as exists for Goffman depends upon the small kindnesses that men bestow upon one another; social systems are fragile little floating islands whose coasts have daily to be shored up and renewed.

Thus, from Goffman's interactionist perspective, 'sturdy social structures drift away into the background' (Gouldner 1971: 380). We might question whether, in attempting to counter structural functionalism's neglect of individuals and their interactions, Goffman has not gone too far in the other direction.

Another possible criticism of Goffman's position is that it presents us with a very dark portrayal of human nature. People are seen as 'tricky, harassed little devils' (Gouldner 1971: 380), always wearing masks in their dealings with others, always worried about their masks slipping and often attempting to expose the masks of others. Irving Zeitlin has remarked upon this bleak view:

> Goffman wants... to transform all of us into agents who expose and discredit others, fearing all the while that we ourselves shall soon be discovered and exposed. In this way, Goffman attributes to the whole of everyday social intercourse a fundamental cynicism.
>
> (1973: 214)

What makes this cynicism difficult to accept in its entirety is the consequences that it would have for individuals: they would simply be unable to sustain a coherent sense of self. Giddens has argued that Goffman takes the metaphor of play-acting too far. If it were really the case that our selves could be reduced to our performances:

> The whole of social life would be, in Sullivan's phrase, a desperate search to put on 'security operations' to salvage a sense of self-esteem in the staging of routines. Those who *do* feel this way characteristically display modes of anxiety of an extreme kind. It is precisely because there is a deep, although generalised, affective involvement in the routines of daily life that actors (agents) do not ordinarily feel themselves to be actors (players), whatever the terminological similarity between the terms.
>
> (Giddens 1984: 125)

Nursing example: nurses' power in interactions with patients

A good example of the use of symbolic interactionism in nursing research can be found in Alistair Hewison's (1995) study of nurse/patient interactions. In this paper, Hewison seeks to uncover the manifestations of power in professional/client encounters. He approaches this issue from the symbolic interactionist perspective that the social world is a process of varied interactions rather than a fixed structure, arguing that 'Social reality is created through interaction and is constantly being negotiated and defined' (Hewison 1995: 76).

Hewison observed interactions between nurses and older women on a 'care of the elderly' ward, using the research technique of participant observation. He identified four different interactional strategies that nurses adopt in order to exercise power over their clients. The first strategy, which he terms 'overt power', sometimes involves nurses openly giving orders or, more subtly, making decisions without asking patients whether they wish to go along with them. In the latter technique, nursing power is the result of 'an expectation on the part of the nurse, and an acceptance on the part of the patient, that the nurse will be in control' (1995: 78–9). Thus, we can see that overt power is not simply a matter of coercion that takes place against the will of the weaker party. In many cases, patients will interpret nurses' position of authority as a legitimate one.

The second strategy used by nurses is termed 'persuasion'. This involves nurses cajoling patients to act in ways with which they are initially unhappy. Hewison notes that interaction involves a lot of negotiation and persuasion in pursuit of common interpretation and understanding. However, this does not mean that all actors in the negotiations have equal power or that their interpretations are regarded as equally valid. Nurses' position within the organisation of health care gives them a privileged position in the negotiating process:

> Nurses, because of their role, are the 'appointed' arbiters of interactional power in the clinical setting: they use persuasion to ensure that patients fall in with their 'understanding' of appropriate behaviour.

> (Hewison 1995: 79)

The third strategy involves 'controlling the agenda'. Hewison argues that this is the most common way in which nurses exert power over elderly patients. Here, the manipulation involves appearing to give patients choice by asking questions but constructing the questions in such a way that the patient has little choice but to go along with what the nurse wants her to do. Thus, the nurse controls the agenda by making it clear to the patient how the situation should be 'properly' interpreted.

The final strategy – 'terms of endearment' – can be used to reinforce the others. In this the nurse interprets her interaction with patients as being similar to that of the relationship between parent and child. If such an interpretation is accepted by patients, the directive and controlling function of nurses is further legitimated in the eyes of both.

Hewison's study gives us a clear insight into the ways in which nurses interpret their relationship with older patients and how they attempt to manipulate the understandings of elderly patients in order to ensure that their behaviour fits with what the nurses feel to be appropriate. However, apart from their manipulation by nurses, there is little mention of how the elderly women observed actively interpreted the world. Hewison is aware of this problem:

> The data presented may seem to suggest that the exercise of power was totally one way. This was not the case and sometimes patients did exert control, but this was a rare occurrence.

> (1995: 80)

The fact that nurses' power was usually successfully applied, and that patients' perspectives had little influence upon subsequent action, might lead us to question whether or not symbolic interactionism can take sufficient account of the significance of coercion in social life. In contrast to Blumer's position that people are not passive recipients of external determining factors but active creators of their own reality, this case seems to show just how much influence external factors can have upon people's behaviour in certain circumstances, irrespective of how they themselves would wish to act. In defence of this sort of criticism, Becker (1963) has argued that interactionism can take account of this facet of social life. He argues that interactionists:

> pay attention to how social actors define each other and their environments. They pay particular attention to differentials in the power to define; in the way one group achieves and uses power to define how other groups will be regarded, understood and treated. Elites... maintain their power as much by controlling how people define the world... as by the use of more primitive forms of power.

> (Becker 1963: 204)

It can be seen that nurses in Hewison's study used both crude methods of control (overt power), and control of definition (persuasion, controlling the agenda and terms of endearment). However, this still begs the question of why elderly patients are not seen as having the capacity for active interpretation. However, there is one transcript in Hewison's paper that may give us a clue to the manner in which elderly people understood their situation:

Pat Alright, sweetie, you want to walk?

Mrs King Whenever you're ready.

Pat No, no, no, no, whenever you're ready, darling.

Mrs King I've always found it so. I have to do as I'm told, I'm 94 next week and I still have to do as I'm told.

(1995: 80)

Here, we can see how this women interpreted her situation as one of inevitable subservience. She had resigned herself to the fact that she had little choice but to accede to the 'requests' of nurses. Nevertheless, it would seem that it was not that nurses gained their power through the way in which they interacted with patients but that they were able to control understandings because they were in possession of institutional power. This objection reflects a central line of criticism of social theories such as interactionism, which argues that, by rejecting the idea that the way in which we act is determined by social structures, interactionists have gone too far in the other direction, failing to give due recognition to the influence of those structures. In philosophical terminology, this objection states that while the understanding of symbolic interaction is necessary for an adequate understanding of the world (and therefore very useful), it may not be sufficient.

Recommended further reading

Probably the best comprehensive text on symbolic interactionism is to be found in Paul Rock's *The Making of Symbolic Interactionism* (1979). For the clearest discussion of the theoretical underpinnings of this approach, Blumer provides a reasonable accessible treatise (1969). Indeed, one of the things about symbolic interactionism is that much of it is written in a straightforward and attractive manner. It is therefore worthwhile going to the horse's mouth, as it were, to explore this strand of sociological thought. In terms of labelling theory, Howard Becker's *Outsiders* (1963) provides a clear theoretical exposition of labelling theory and some juicy substantive examples, using the cases of marihuana smokers and dance musicians. Finally, Erving Goffman's *Stigma* (1968b [1963]) is a short and accessible book, well worth the read.

6 Phenomenology and ethnomethodology

Introduction

This chapter will discuss two separate but closely related areas of social theory. The first area to be addressed is that of phenomenology. This will commence with a review of the ideas of the founding father of phenomenology, Edmund Husserl. It will then go on to discuss how Alfred Schutz combined these ideas with the work of Max Weber in order to develop a social phenomenology. This examination of Schutz is followed by the nursing example of Janice Morse *et al.*'s 'The phenomenology of comfort' (1994). The chapter then moves on to review the efforts of Harold Garfinkel and other ethnomethodologists to operationalise social phenomenology into a practical research strategy. The chapter concludes with a nursing example of the use of ethnomethodology, in the form of Len Bowers' (1992b) study of the community psychiatric nurse in the patient's home.

Husserl and phenomenology

The inauguration of the modern phenomenological movement can be found in the work of Edmund Husserl (1859–1938). Husserl wrote a number of seminal texts, the most notable probably being *Logical Investigations* (1970 [1900]). The starting point of Husserl's philosophy was what he saw as the inadequacies of the theories of knowledge, most importantly scientific knowledge, that were current when he was writing.

The dominant theory of knowledge at the time was that of positivism – the doctrine asserting that the only valid form of knowledge was scientific knowledge. One of the crucial assumptions of positivism was that of 'subject–object dualism'. This involved the belief that it was possible (and indeed essential) to separate the 'external' world, which consists of 'objects' that we can know about, from the 'internal' world of the 'subjective' consciousness, which receives knowledge of the external world. For positivism, the route to valid knowledge lay in the implementation of methods and procedures that controlled and standardised human subjectivity, so that its representations of the 'objective' world would not be influenced by personal idiosyncrasies. Thus, for example, the strict rules of procedure that apply to experiments are there to ensure that the results produced by those experiments will not be influenced by the character or prejudices of the experimenter but will solely reflect the nature of the object or process that the experimenter is studying.

This theory of science has had considerable influence upon our everyday assumptions about knowledge. Thus, when we wish to brand a person's ideas as little more than opinion and prejudice, we describe them as being 'subjective'. In contrast, when we wish to portray our own ideas as being wholly correct, we claim that we are being 'objective'.

The crucial point here is the positivist claim that there is a world of 'facts' out there that are what they are, irrespective of what people think about them. The role of the human subject is merely to apprehend those facts as faithfully as possible.

For Husserl, this conception of the generation of knowledge was fatally flawed because it failed to recognise the active component of human consciousness. He argued that the very notion of an objective world, distinct and divorced from the human thinker, is itself a product of the human mind. While positivists took this ordering of the world as fundamental, Husserl argued that it was the result of conceptual judgements of the human mind. More fundamental than these conceptual judgements that objectify the world are the lived experiences prior to those judgements, which are subsequently ordered and categorised.

Before the world becomes an object that we know, it is an experience that we live (Kearney 1994). If science is to be adequately founded, we are required to uncover the process by which human consciousness gives meaning to lived experience. This is why Husserl calls his philosophy 'phenomenology', the word having its root in the Greek for 'appearance' – his aim was to get to the very roots of knowledge by uncovering how the world first *appears* to the human consciousness. The task was therefore to strip back the study of knowledge to its very basics, to abandon all assumptions (scientific or otherwise) about the nature of the world, so that we might once again see it in a fresh light as it really is in our lived experience.

This is not to say that Husserl was a naïve idealist who believed that everything was in the mind. For him, meaning was neither in the mind alone nor in the world alone, but in the relationship between the two. On the one hand, the world is disclosed by consciousness. On the other, consciousness is conscious of something other than itself – the world. Even this is to overplay the distinction between mind and world for, as Husserl's pupil Martin Heidegger (1962 [1927]) argued, human existence and consciousness is a matter of 'being-in-the-world'.

In his later works, Husserl became ever more convinced of the folly of disciplines such as psychology, which claim to be able to gain an objective understanding of what goes on in the minds of human beings. He argued that when we use objective science in our attempts to understand people, we fossilise living experience, turning consciousness into a thing. Husserl, as a Jew living in Germany in the 1930s, was acutely aware of the dangers that resulted from the categorisation of human beings as objects. In the conclusion of a lecture he gave in 1935 while in exile from Nazi Germany, entitled *Philosophy and the Crisis of Modern European Man* (in Husserl 1965), Husserl made a passionate plea for a return to reason, a reason that does not objectify humanity, treating the person as nothing more than another component of the natural world (an approach he terms 'naturalism') but which accepts the human spirit as a fundamental and active entity:

> The collapse of a rational culture does not lie in the essence of rationalism itself but only in its exteriorization, its absorption in naturalism and objectivism. The crisis of European existence can end only in one of two ways: in the ruin of Europe alienated from its rational sense of life, fallen into a barbarian hatred of spirit; or in the rebirth of Europe in the spirit of philosophy, through a heroism of reason that will definitively overcome naturalism.
>
> (1935, cited by Kearney 1994: 24)

From a general philosophical point of view, it is not hard to see how Husserl's approach to knowledge might appeal to those who wish to engage in holistic care. Husserl's work provides a powerful philosophical base for the contention that clients should not be treated as objects but as active, thinking individuals. It is therefore not surprising that Husserl is oft cited as a theoretical base by those nurses who wish to approach examination of practice from a phenomenological perspective. Unfortunately, Husserl's philosophy cannot be so easily adapted to practical empirical research. While, as we have seen, his ontology (theory of what exists) is highly compatible with new nursing concerns, his epistemology (theory of what we can know about what exists) is less so. Husserl has very definite ideas about the way in which we should go about gaining phenomenological understanding, one which is highly individualised.

Given that they are not of direct use for nurses wishing to examine practice, I will not describe in great detail the rather convoluted and complex methods recommended by Husserl. At the core of his method is individual introspection, centring around the person examining her own thoughts. The first stage of this introspection involves the 'bracketing' of all the presuppositions that we have in our 'natural attitude'; included in these presuppositions is our assumption that the outside world exists independently of our consciousness. Through this bracketing, Husserl argues that we are able to recover the presuppositionless world of our immediate thoughts. Once the phenomenologist has achieved this stage, the next step is to play around with these thoughts, testing their possibilities and limits. Husserl (1960 [1929]) uses the example of a table, arguing that the aim of the phenomenological method at this point was to imagine the various possibilities of table shape, colour, size and so on, until the phenomenologist managed to boil down her conception of a table to its essential attributes, getting rid of any superfluous aspects. This may sound a bit off the wall, but this search for essences is part of a long philosophical tradition stretching back to Plato. The next stage of phenomenological analysis is to reflect critically upon the essences that have emerged from the process of the free play of immediate thoughts. Finally, the phenomenologist records and describes the previous stages of analysis, contributing to the archive of phenomenological knowledge.

The problem with Husserl's method, even if we accept it as a viable way in which to gain understanding, is that it is hard to imagine it being a great help to someone wishing to understand the everyday world of nursing practice. In short, because Husserl's method is introspection, it cannot act as a guide for empirical research. To find such a guide, we need to turn to another phenomenological thinker, Alfred Schutz (1899–1959), who is accredited with introducing phenomenology to the discipline of sociology. However, before examining Schutz's ideas in detail, we need to make a digression and return to the theories of Max Weber. The reason for this is that, along with Husserl's phenomenology, Weber's conception of the sociological task provides the starting point for Schutz's phenomenological sociology.

Weber and *Verstehen*

For Max Weber, the focus of sociology should be not on social structures or laws but on the social actions of thinking human beings. Weber was insistent that the fundamental unit of analysis for sociologists should be the individual person. The reason for this insistence was that human beings (and only human beings) are capable of meaningful action.

The importance of the human capacity to engage in meaningful action lies in the fact that this capacity differentiates them from everything else in the world. Molecules, plants, rocks, or whatever, are incapable of thought and are therefore subject to the physical, chemical and biological laws of the universe. When a plant grows towards the sun, it is not because it has decided that this is the direction that it would most like to go in but rather because its chemical make-up ensures that it is subject to the law of phototropism. When a rock falls from a cliff face unto a beach, it is not because it fancies a change of scenery but because it has been subjected to the combined laws of liquid thermodynamics and gravity. In contrast, the reasons why a human being goes to the beach to lie in the sun is that she has feels a bit pallid, remembers the pleasure of daydreaming on warm sand, realises that she has got a day off, that the weather forecast is good, that it won't matter too much if the grass doesn't get cut for another week, and, as a result, comes to the decision to grab her swimming costume and head for the coast.

According to Weber, the first error of positivist sociologists such as Comte was that they treated human beings in the same fashion as rocks or plants, portraying them as puppets whose actions were directed according to anonymous laws rather than as beings capable of making their own minds up. The second error that he accused them of committing was to ascribe to social structures themselves the capacity to engage in meaningful actions. Weber's objection here was that, because social structures or institutions do not have minds, it is an error to treat them as if they are volitional actors:

> for sociological purposes there is no such thing as a collective personality which 'acts'. When reference is made in a sociological context to a state, a nation, a corporation, a family or an army corps, or to similar collectivities, what is meant is ... only a certain kind of actual or possible social actions of individual persons.
>
> (Weber 1968a: 14)

For Weber, the focus of sociology should be upon what he termed 'social action', which he defined as *those actions that are meaningfully oriented to other human beings*. As will be seen from the discussion above, the word 'meaningful' is important here because it involves the assertion that sociology should be concerned with the motives and understandings of individual actors in their relations with others rather than with the mechanisms that make them act in certain ways.

In rejecting the notion that our actions are determined by inexorable outside forces or laws, Weber was privileging the notion of choice. We are constantly faced with alternative courses of action and, as a consequence, with decisions on which courses of action we are going to take in preference to others. The decisions that we make, given that they are not determined by external social forces, will be largely based upon our perceptions and understanding of the situations in which we find ourselves. As a consequence, in order to explain social actions, the sociologist is required to gain an understanding of how the social actor perceived the possible options that she had and how she assessed the benefits and pitfalls of each option in order to come to a decision to act in a certain way.

Thus, the task of sociology, according to Weber (1964), is to try to gain an interpretative understanding of social action in order to arrive at an explanation of why that action happened and what its effects were. This is where the theory of *Verstehen*, which is German for understanding, comes in. The aim of the *Verstehen* method of sociological enquiry is to explain social action in terms of a 'sequence of motivation, the understanding of which can be treated as an explanation of the actual course of behaviour' (Weber 1968a: 10–11). To do that, the sociologist has to discover or reconstruct the understandings, motives, constraints and opportunities experienced by the social actor prior to her action. Thus, for example, from a Weberian point of view, a time-and-motion analysis of nursing activity that discovers that nurses spend 15 per cent of their time sitting on patients' beds would tell us very little. In order to understand this form of social action, the researcher would also need to discover the 'sequence of motivations' that led nurses to sit on beds, and this sequence may well be different in different instances of behaviour that on the surface look exactly the same. Thus, the sociologist would need to discover, for each occasion on which she observes a nurse sitting on a bed, whether the nurse is doing so because she is tired of cleaning the sluice and wants to rest her legs, whether she is discussing the patient's worries about the effects that a myocardial infarction will have upon her daily life after discharge, or whether she is asking the patient to choose her dinner from the hospital's menu.

To summarise Weber's position, the task of sociology is to gain an understanding (*Verstehen*) of social action. This can only be done by understanding the subjective meanings held by social actors, meanings that provide actors with the motivation to act in the ways in which they do.

Schutz and phenomenological sociology

Weber's work on *Verstehen* provided the basis for Alfred Schutz's social phenomenology. While Schutz was highly supportive of the direction in which Weber had tried to take sociology, he argued that Weber's model was far too vague, leaving many crucial questions unanswered. As Schutz noted in the preface to his seminal work, *The Phenomenology of the Social World*:

> The present study is based on an intensive concern of many years' duration with the theoretical writings of Max Weber. During this time I became convinced that while Weber's approach was correct and that he had determined conclusively the proper starting point of the philosophy of the social sciences, nevertheless his analyses did not go deeply enough to lay the foundations on which alone many important problems

of the human sciences could be solved. Above all, Weber's central concept of subjective meaning calls for a thoroughgoing analysis. As Weber left this concept, it was little more than a heading for a number of important problems which he did not examine in detail.

(1972: xxvii)

At the core of Schutz's dissatisfaction with Weber was what he saw as the latter's failure to state clearly the essential attributes of understanding (*Verstehen*), of subjective meaning or of social action. In order to deal with these central concepts with the rigour and exactitude that Schutz felt they deserved, it was necessary to turn to Husserl. The key idea that Schutz adopted from Husserl was his assertion that what looks to us like the natural ordering of the world is in fact the result of conceptual judgements of our mind. Schutz echoes Husserl's castigation of positivism and 'naturalism' (the treatment of humans as if they are merely natural objects, subject without choice to cause and effect), by pointing out that to adopt such positions is to take as given that which is constructed by human consciousness. In relation to the study of society, this leads to a failure to account for the way in which social reality is constructed and maintained as a subjective phenomenon. Moreover, Schutz argued that humans do not attach meaning to the world in an individual manner. Rather, our phenomenological understandings of the world are shared with, and reinforced by, other members of society: they are 'intersubjective'. Indeed, it is only on such a basis that we are able to communicate with each other. In attaching such importance to the notion of intersubjectivity, Schutz's approach is considerably more sociological than Husserl's. While Husserl had actually introduced the term 'intersubjective', he did so late in his career, and he maintained a rather ambivalent attitude toward it.

According to Schutz, we approach the world on the basis of a stock of common-sense knowledge, much of which is passed on to us as children but which is constantly being modified and refined on the basis of our experiences and interactions in the world. We see the world through 'typifications', or conceptual frameworks, into which we slot the events and activities that we experience in order to make sense of them. For the most part, we are not consciously aware of these typifications (or 'recipes' as he also called them). Rather, in our 'natural attitude', we take it for granted that they consist of the facts of life and assume that others around us see these facts of life in the same way. So, for example, when a person is being admitted to hospital and sees a woman in a white trouser suit, she attaches to this sight a number of implicit assumptions about that person and the role she plays. For example, the patient may not be overly alarmed if the person takes her to a bed, draws the curtains round and asks her to undress (whereas she might well be alarmed if the person was wearing a uniform that we associate with the fire service or the police). Nor would the patient be particularly put out if the person broke the normal codes of bodily space by telling her that they wished to take her pulse and gently taking hold of her wrist. Instead, according to the recipe under which they are working, she might accept that the purpose of this intimacy is to ascertain her pulse rate and quality in order to assist with diagnosis and thus to contribute to the healing of the physical ills that brought her into the hospital in the first place. Once again, we do not have such a typification of the role of bank-tellers and would therefore find such an instance of touching as 'unnatural'.

Schutz's criticism of the social science of his day was that sociologists failed to rise above the typifications of the society in which they lived, taking them as part of an objective reality and regarding their role as explaining that objective reality. In contrast, Schutz argued that the contribution of phenomenology to sociology was to point to the social construction of the natural attitude. The task of phenomenological sociology was not to explain the world 'out there' but to uncover how that world was constructed through the actions and understandings of social actors. In this sense, Schutz's ideas owe a great deal to Husserl's technique of 'bracketing' the natural attitude, in that he regarded it the responsibility of social scientists to pull back from the natural attitudes of the society around them and to act as if they were strangers to society, taking nothing for granted and questioning how the 'recipes' that people use in order to get through their lives are formulated and accepted.

While Schutz's view of the way in which the social scientist should approach her subject matter has a considerable amount in common with Husserl's approach, there are also major differences in his approach. The most important of these is that, while Husserl regarded the natural attitude of the 'lived world' as a barrier to true understanding, for Schutz, understanding how the natural attitude was constituted was the prime purpose of the social scientist. What for Husserl was a diversion was for Schutz a fascination. Indeed, while he went out of his way to praise the intellectual innovations of Husserl, Schutz was quite firm that Husserl's method of 'transcendental phenomenology' could not be used as a basis for social scientific enquiry:

> We may say that the empirical social sciences will find their true foundation not in transcendental phenomenology, but in the constitutive phenomenology of the natural attitude. Husserl's signal contribution to the social sciences consists neither in his unsuccessful attempt to solve the problem of the constitution of the transcendental intersubjectivity within the reduced egological sphere [that is, the method of individual introspection to uncover pure consciousness], nor in his unclarified notion of empathy as the foundation of understanding... but rather in the wealth of his analyses pertinent to the problems of the Lebenswelt [lifeworld] and designed to be developed into a philosophical anthropology.
>
> (Schutz 1962: 149)

The central aim of Schutzian phenomenology is to address the problems of the 'lifeworld' – the world constructed by the natural attitude, which forms our 'intuitive environment', in which 'we, as human beings among fellow-beings, experience culture and society, take a stand with regard to their objects, are influenced by them and act upon them' (Schutz 1966: 116).

Nursing example: the phenomenology of comfort

Numerous examples of nursing research into practice using phenomenology as a theoretical foundation could be cited. Here, I choose one that is co-written by a pioneer of qualitative nursing research, Janice Morse. In at least one important respect, 'The phenomenology of comfort' (Morse *et al.* 1994) is typical of nursing approaches to phenomenology, in that it does not explicitly base itself on the writings of phenomenological theorists such as Husserl, Heidegger or Schutz. Instead, it is founded on an operationalisation of phenomenology designed for use by practical researchers (van Manen 1990). Morse *et al.* construct their research into the phenomenon of comfort using the seven activities of research outlined by van Manen:

turning to the nature of lived experience; exploring the lived experience in all its aspects while reflecting on essential themes of the experience that give it its special significance; writing and rewriting to capture the fullness and richness of this experience; maintaining a strong orientation to the fundamental questions of the project, and balancing the research context by considering the parts and the wholes.

(Morse *et al*. 1994: 190)

Morse *et al*. begin their examination of comfort by noting that it is an extremely difficult phenomenon to examine or even to express:

On the one hand the experience of comfort is difficult to describe because it is pre-reflexive; a way of being that is beyond physical or mental awareness... on the other hand, because we more easily speak of our pains, problems and weaknesses, it is hard to find a language to describe comfort states.

(Morse *et al*. 1994: 190)

To put this into Schutzian terms, because comfort is usually embedded in our natural attitude, we take it for granted, and it is only when that natural attitude is disrupted that we become consciously aware of comfort as something that is missing. Comfort, ironically, only becomes recognisable when we no longer enjoy it.

It is through the medium of discomfort that Morse *et al*. seek to analyse the nature of comfort and how nurses can contribute to its recovery. They show how this process is essentially a negative one, involving the person forgetting the discomfort that is generated by the sick body. It is a 'freeing from the bondage' of the experience of sickness or disability. Morse *et al*. identify nine different but connected states of discomfort, of which I will summarise five. The first state is that of the 'dis-eased body'. Here, the onset of symptoms progressively alters a person's experience of her body, with all the annoyance, irritation and often unbearability that they entail. Morse *et al*. argue that a person in this state of dis-ease primarily requires knowledge about what is wrong with them and what can be done to help. Moreover, the experience of dis-ease will be more effectively ameliorated if nurses work *with* the person, affirming their subjectivity, rather than simply doing things *to* them.

The second state is termed the 'disobedient body'. Here, the person experiences a loss of control over functions of her body, which generates experiences of apprehension, frustration and embarrassment. While it may not be possible to eradicate the symptoms that have caused loss of control, an important role for the nurse is ensuring that the impact of those symptoms upon the person's everyday life is minimised. This can be done through the nurse supporting the person's efforts to control the situation in which she finds herself and to regain independence.

The third category is the 'vulnerable body', which involves the dread of painful experiences and the feelings of vulnerability associated with such dread. In order to minimise the experience of dread, Morse *et al.* argue that nurses need to be patient and sensitive to the fact that those who feel vulnerable require protection until such times as they regain trust in their bodies and their care.

Another cause for discomfort comes from the experience of the 'violated body', in which health care procedures invade the person's private world, leading to feelings of embarrassment and loss of dignity. Morse *et al.* identify a number of strategies that people use to find comfort in the face of such violation. One is mental detachment from their bodies. Morse *et al.*'s observation that 'Sometimes the presence of and connection with a nurse is important in facilitating the objectification of the body' (1994: 192) is interesting, not only because there is much sense in their argument that nurses can help to refocus attention away from the embarrassments of the exposed or violated body. We might also think back to Husserl's strong opposition to the whole notion of objectification and note that, in some circumstances, the treatment of human bodies as objects is, paradoxically, a very humane approach to take.

The next experience is that of the 'enduring body'. This involves those unfortunate people for whom there is no escape from pain. In such a situation, all else that was taken for granted in life loses its relevance as the total presence of pain dominates consciousness. Morse *et al.* argue that one way in which people try to gain the strength of endurance is to refocus their attention away from the experience of pain. The task of the nurse is therefore to aid this process of refocusing and, when this is not possible, to aid the person's endurance of the most painful experiences by 'talking them through each moment' (1994: 192).

In working through these and other themes, Morse *et al.* do not rely on 'scientific' data to make their points; rather, they cite the feelings of people who have experienced these states, as expressed in their own words. Thus, for example, in discussing the experience of the violated body, they quote the feelings of a patient in that situation:

> I would have to put up a little wall so that I could become a little bit colder, a little bit harder so their words that they were talking to each other or things that could hurt me, couldn't penetrate me.

> (Morse *et al.* 1994: 192)

The key point here is that the phenomenological researcher does not examine 'objective' facts about illness but rather seeks to uncover the subjective meanings that illness has for the person who is experiencing it, or, in Schutzian terms, to address the problems of the lifeworld. Nor is it simply a matter for the researcher; Morse *et al.* argue that striving for phenomenological understanding should be a core part of clinical nursing practice, noting that, as nurses, we need to be sensitive to the strategies that people adopt to maintain or restore their phenomenological orientation to the world in the face of discomfort. Nurses need to recognise the states of discomfort that patients experience and to assist them in their attempts to recover comfort to the greatest degree that their circumstances allow.

Ethnomethodology

As I noted at the start of my discussion of 'The phenomenology of comfort', Morse *et al.* do not refer to phenomenological theorists such as Husserl of Schutz in their paper. Instead, they look to a commentator who has attempted to adapt those ideas for use in practical research. There are good reasons for this second-hand approach to social phenomenology, in that even Schutz, with his desire to bring Husserl's rather rarefied ideas down to earth so that they could be used in the understanding of the issues of daily life, maintained a high philosophical approach that did not deal fully with how phenomenology might be practically applied. The most concerted attempt to pin this philosophy down to the practicalities of social research has been made by Howard Garfinkel (1984 [1967]) through his development of ethnomethodology.

'Ethnomethodology' is a neologism coined by Garfinkel. This rather daunting piece of jargon is probably most easily understood by breaking it down into its constituent syllables; it involves the study (ology) of people's (ethno) methods of knowing about and creating social order (method). Garfinkel's approach to sociological research starts with his acceptance of the phenomenological critique of positivism. For positivism, there is an objective world out there, and the aim of science is to gain knowledge that corresponds as closely as possible to that objective reality. This approach is known as the correspondence theory of truth. The point of the scientific method is that the procedures it involves ensure that the appearance of objective reality in scientific discourse corresponds as closely as possible to the external object being studied. In line with Husserl and Schutz, Garfinkel rejects this division between the object and its perception by the human mind. In contrast to the correspondence theory, Garfinkel posits what he calls a 'congruence view of reality', in which the 'concrete object' and the 'perceived object' are synonymous and interchangeable (Benson and Hughes 1983). In other words, our perception of the world 'out there' *is* the world out there. Thus, for Garfinkel, there is no such thing as external social reality that orders our actions in the world. The order that we perceive in the world around us is just that – our perception. Indeed, we put a lot of energy into making sense of the world, of constituting order out of the events that we experience. The aim of ethnomethodology is to uncover the methods that people use to create such order. As a consequence, the focus of ethnomethodology is not on large-scale or unusual events but on the mundane activities in which people engage during their daily lives:

> Ethnomethodology asks *'How* do people *do* things?' How do they accomplish tasks and how do they make their accomplishments known to others as well as to themselves. How do they *account* for what they do? And how does the very accounting – or the methods they use for making their activities visible as rational, commonplace, everyday activities – feed back into the situation to make the activity *real* for the interactants?
>
> (Morris 1977: 39)

In their interrogation of these questions, ethnomethodologists have developed a number of theories about the everyday construction of social reality. First, following directly from Schutz's notion of recipes, is the identification of 'background expectancies', or common-sense assumptions about how the world is ordered. In order to demonstrate the strength of these assumptions, one of the most favoured forms of research in ethnomethodology has been the 'breaching experiment', in which the researcher breaches the background expectancies in a given social situation. Thus, for example, Garfinkel sent his students home to act as if they were lodgers. This new approach to their parents, unsurprisingly, caused considerable consternation, and the assumption by a number of parents that their children were ill. The point of such an experiment was to demonstrate that parents had very well-worked out expectations of what their social role and the social role of their children should be, expectations that the parents would never otherwise think to question because they were regarded as 'natural' or 'common sense'. You might think that such an experiment is rather trivial and demonstrates only the obvious point that if people behave significantly differently from their usual behaviour without explanation, those around them will tend to be perplexed. If you do think this trivial, you are in the company of a goodly number of commentators (for example, Craib 1984).

Another concept developed by ethnomethodologists is that of 'reflexivity'. This is the assertion that people's description of their actions and the social world around them is at the same time the creation of that world. This process often involves what Garfinkel terms the 'documentary method', which is in essence an exercise in circular reasoning: we select certain particular aspects of the social world and see in them evidence of an underlying pattern, and then we use the same sorts of instance to justify our assertion of the existence of such patterning. Thus, the instance is explained by the pattern, and the pattern is justified by the instance. Take the example of a nurse trying to persuade a reluctant older patient to have a bath. Despite exercising all her persuasive powers, Mr Byrne refuses to enter the water. The nurse puts this down to his being Irish and therefore averse to hygiene (the instance being explained by the pattern). A couple of days later, she is sitting in a bar, chatting to friends about life in general, and the topic gets round to immigration, with which she does not agree. When challenged about this, she argues that her opposition is based upon the fact that immigrants lower

British cultural standards. She illustrates this assertion with the example of the dirty Irish. Once again she is challenged on what a friend regards as racism. She defends herself by saying, 'I'm just stating facts. You get to see things when you are a nurse. A few days ago I spent half an hour trying to persuade an old Paddy to have a bath and he would have none of it. And that's only one example; they are all the same' (the pattern being justified by the instance). Thus, what we have here is not an external social structure of racism but a racist mental construct in the head of the nurse. I should add that this begs the question of the effect that this has upon Mr Byrne. Is it simply a mental construct of his that some British people with whom he comes into contact treat him as a second-class citizen on the grounds that they have mental constructs that place Irish people in such a position? Or is he the victim of a real racism that is external to him and exists independently of whether or not he sees it that way? After all, he may think that he, as an individual, is not very personable, and this is the reason why some English people treat him with a degree of disdain, but that does not negate the fact that the nurse regarded him in a racist fashion. The inability to take full cognisance of external structures of power has been identified as one of the significant weaknesses of ethnomethodology (Gouldner 1971).

The notion of the documentary method might give the impression that we develop fixed attitudes about what we see as the social patterns around us and stick to them regardless of our context. However, this is not how ethnomethodologists see things. Instead, they regard the construction of social reality as a very fragile thing that requires considerable practical effort on the part of society's members to keep that social order real in their heads. It will be remembered that the basic point of the ethnomethodological notion of reflexivity is that the description and creation of the social world are synonymous. Placing such emphasis on description brings language to the fore; after all, it is through language that we describe things. Relying on the philosophy of the later Wittgenstein (1953) (the word 'later' is used because early in his career, Wittgenstein was a positivist), ethnomethodologists argue that there are no fixed and unequivocal rules for the use of language. Instead, they argue that the meaning that a word has will depend upon the context within which it is being used. This is obviously the case for some statements, notably those including pronouns such as 'you' or 'him', the meaning of which will depend upon the particular person being referred to. However, ethnomethodologists argue that all language is 'indexical' (that is, it is indexed, or linked to its context). That being the case, people's construction of social order will differ depending on the situation in which they find themselves.

Even what might be thought of as fairly rigid rules of social behaviour are subject to what Garfinkel calls the *et cetera* rule, which allows people to break the initial rule in certain circumstances. So, for example, it may be a rule in a coronary care ward that all cardiac drugs have to be prescribed by a physician. However, the *et cetera* rule might be brought into play by a nurse if, when she comes to a patient with some glyceryl trinitrate in order to relieve his angina, the patient points out that that particular drug, in his 12 years' experience of angina, has never done anything for him. If he goes on to request his favoured drug, nifedipine, the nurse is unlikely to refuse to give it to him on the grounds that there is not a physician about to prescribe it. Thus, the initial rule about prescription has been broken by an *et cetera* rule that has been generated by the nurse's perception of the particular social context in which she finds herself. The import of practical actions such as this is that generalised sociological commentaries on the power relations between doctors and nurses, for example, which state that one of the buttresses of medical power is exclusive control over prescription, fail to take account of the day-to-day activities of nurses, which are far more flexible and complex than such generalisations can take account of. The central point being made by ethnomethodologists in relation to the indexicality of the social world is that sociological attempts to view that world as objective and uniform will be inadequate. Instead, the sociologist is restricted to understanding the practical accomplishments of actors in specific contexts.

To sum up, the focus of ethnomethodology is on the common-sense activities of ordinary members of society in their everyday lives, a topic that most other branches of sociology take for granted (Swingewood 1991). This world is reflexive in that people's way of knowing and accounting for their social situation also involves the creation of that social situation. It is also indexical, in that the meaning that the social world has for people is context bound.

Nursing example: the ethnomethodology of home visiting

An illuminating use of ethnomethodology in nursing research, which is accompanied by a paper outlining the theory of ethnomethodology (Bowers 1992a), can be found in Len Bowers' 'Ethnomethodology II: a study of the community psychiatric nurse in the patient's home' (Bowers 1992b). As the title suggests, the paper involves the examination of how the social actors involved socially construct home visits.

The interest of these social encounters lies in the tensions that they involve, most notably for nurses. On the one hand, most community psychiatric nurses (CPNs) come from a hospital background. As a result, the typifications that they have about the appropriate forms of interaction between nurse and patient are coloured by this setting, in which the nurse enjoys a considerable degree of power and control. On the other hand, the social interaction involved in visiting people's homes carries with it its own set of typifications involving the appropriate behaviour of a visitor towards her host. These typifications form 'the backdrop against which the actions of the participants are judged by each other and made meaningful' (Bowers 1992b: 77). Their most significant effect is that they radically alter the asymmetry of the power relationships between nurse and patient that would pertain in the setting of a health care institution.

Given these tensions, the questions Bowers asks are how nurses and patients accomplish the social task of home visiting and how they account for what they do. The first thing he notes in relation to the issue of power and control is the power that playing host confers upon the patient:

> The dominance of the patient in his own home is demonstrated in several ways. From the moment the CPN knocks at the patient's door much of the initiative stays with the patient. He takes the lead. It is the patient who decides where in the house the visit is to take place... The dominance and initiative of the patient is clearly recognized by CPNs, and they formulate it in various ways. They indicate that the home is the patient's domain and territory, that the patient is the boss and is in charge.
>
> (Bowers 1992b: 75)

One of the consequences of this dominance was that requests that could have been made with ease in a clinical setting became extremely difficult to manage in the patient's home. Thus, for example, CPNs reported considerable difficulties in relation to televisions being switched on during visits. While they all found this a distraction, none of them took it upon themselves to turn it off. To do so, under the typifications of the visitor/guest relationship, would be seen by both actors as being extremely rude. While some felt able to ask the patient to turn the television off, others felt that even this was too much of a refraction of the etiquette of the situation and compromised with a request to turn the volume down in the hope that the patient would take up the cue and turn the television off altogether, thus maintaining the mutual construction of appropriate behaviour. One CPN could not even go this far, reporting that he could not ask, on the grounds that if patients wanted the television off in order to concentrate on the visit, they would turn it off themselves without prompting.

The problem for CPNs was that visits to patients' homes were not just that – they were also health care interactions in which nurses felt they required to exert a degree of influence and control. Their task was to do this without violating the mutual typifications associated with home visiting: 'The CPNs find that they need to develop methods of exerting pressure on their patients without contravening normative visit behaviour' (Bowers 1992b: 77).

Two approaches were taken to this problem. The first was to couch attempts to control the situation in the language of politeness. Thus, rather than giving direct instructions, the nurses would suggest, give guidance and negotiate. This sort of strategy was acceptable because it left the final decision of whether to comply or not with the patients, allowing them to refuse or circumvent the request if they so desired.

The second approach involved a mutual acceptance that there were some areas of the patients' lives that were clearly within the remit of psychiatric care and others that were not. Thus, while whether the television should remain on during the visit was seen as lying solely within the prerogative of the patient, issues surrounding medication and hospital attendance were regarded as areas in which the CPN had the right, through an appeal to superior knowledge and expertise, to give directions.

The importance of Bowers' study lies in its highlighting of the significance of mundane, everyday interactions in the lives of nurses and patients. It shows just how sophisticated are the accomplishments of actors in constructing the social meaning of those interactions on the basis of the mutual typifications they have about the sorts of behaviour that are permissible and required. The power of ethnomethodology is its capacity to shed light upon those interpersonal actions and reactions in which we constantly involve ourselves but which, by their very nature, we rarely fully reflect upon.

Recommended further reading

Neither phenomenology not ethnomethodology makes for easy reading. The former tends to be described in a rather lugubrious Germanic style, while the latter is bogged down with American neologisms. Thomas Luckmann has edited a volume of readings entitled *Phenomenology and Sociology* (1978), although much of this material falls into the category of 'difficult'. One reasonably accessible sociological treatment of phenomenology is to be found in Berger and Luckmann's *The Social Construction of Everyday Life* (1967). While I have not discussed this book here, it represents a highly important contribution to sociological theory. A more critical approach to phenomenology can be found in Robert Gorman's *The Dual Vision* (1977), which entails an examination of the tensions generated by Schutz's attempt to marry Husserl and Weber.

In relation to ethnomethodology, two texts stand out as being as clear as is possible, given the nature of their subject matter. These are John Heritage's *Garfinkel and Ethnomethodology* (1984) and Benson and Hughes' *The Perspective of Ethnomethodology* (1983).

PART III

Bringing it all together

As the title of this part suggests, the two chapters contained in it will address the ideas of theorists who have attempted to overcome the divisions that have emerged between different schools of social theory. In Chapter 7, we will examine, among its other concerns, critical theory's attempt to synthesise the interpretations of capitalism and Western science posited by Marx, Weber and the phenomenologists. In Chapter 8, we will look at theories that seek to take due account of both social structures and individual actions. However, before going any further, it is necessary to make some comments about the latter debate. While the previous section dealt in depth with theorists who asserted the importance of social action, we have not paid so much attention to those who place their emphasis on social structures. This needs to be rectified.

In Part II, we looked at approaches that regarded individuals, their interpretations of the world and their interactions within it as the fundamental subject matter of social analysis. As such, these theories were in contrast to some of those examined in Part I, which involved the assumption that there was something more to society than just the individuals in it. Durkheim, in particular, took such a position, to the point where he argued that 'individuals are a more a product of common life than its determinant' (1964:18). Durkheim (1938) identified what he termed 'social facts', collective entities such as the family, or religion, which he saw as real things because of their capacity to influence the patterns of individual conduct. He argued that social facts 'structure' human actions; in other words, they act as external forces to regulate and constrain those actions. This sort of approach is described as structuralism.

In Chapter 2, the discussion on Durkheim took a specific turn, concentrating more on the development of his functionalism than his structuralism. We would therefore do well to take another look at structuralism in order to set the stage for the next two chapters, particularly Chapter 8. I wish to make mention of two key structuralist thinkers – Ferdinand Saussure (1857–1913) and Louis Althusser (1918–90).

Saussure was a linguist who argued that the system of language is far more important than the actual utterances we make. He published very little in his life, achieving only posthumous fame following the publication of his lectures, gathered up from notes taken by his students, in a book called the *Course in General Linguistics* (1974 [1916]) In this work, he provided a number of reasons why the structure of language should be given primacy. I will briefly mention three. First, individual utterances can only make sense if they are part of a linguistic system: we need to know the rules of the game before we can play. Second, utterances are defined not in their own terms but in terms of their relations to other concepts. Our words do not stand alone; when we speak about things, we are always implicitly comparing and contrasting them to other linguistic concepts. Third, the absorption of language is a condition of being able to think. While people can decide to accept or reject particular beliefs, they cannot throw off the system of meaning that the language they have learned imposes upon their thoughts. Apart from his influence on linguistics, Saussure has also had a considerable effect upon a wide range of disciplines, in which various theorists have accepted his notion that general structures are more important than specific instances. Thus, in anthropology, we have the work of Claude Lévi-Strauss; in literary criticism, Roland Barthes; in psychoanalysis, Jacques Lacan; and in Marxism, Louis Althusser – to name but a few. What all of these theorists have in common can be summed up in their assertion of the 'death of the subject':

'the death of the subject' is the slogan most closely associated with structuralism. 'Subject' means what I have referred to as agency, action and persons. The idea being attacked is that people are the authors of their thoughts and actions. It is assumed instead that people are the puppets of their ideas, and their actions are determined not by choice and decision but are the outcome of the underlying structure of ideas. If for example, I am a Christian, I do not speak about Christianity, rather Christianity speaks through me; some structuralists reach the extreme of saying that people do not speak but rather they are spoken (by the under-lying structure of the language), that they do not read books but are 'read' by books. They do not create societies but are created by societies.

(Craib 1984: 109)

In the 1960s and 70s, structuralism enjoyed great influence over Marxist thinking, largely due to the figure of Louis Althusser (Althusser and Balibar 1970), who regarded the belief in the importance of the subject as nothing more than a bourgeois myth. Althusser took a selective approach to Marx's writings, regarding his early work on such matters as alienation (with its obvious concentration on the concerns of the human subject) as immature. In contrast, he argued that Marx's later 'scientific' phase was a far more fruitful avenue of departure. As we shall see in the next chapter, critical theorists take precisely the opposite approach, emphasising the importance of the early, humanist, Marx and crit-icising the scientific pretensions of his later work for its potential to reduce human beings to the status of manipulable objects.

Marx (1946) argued that people are largely moulded by their social environments. Althusser extrapolates from this to argue that there can be no account of what people are like prior to society. It is society that constructs the individual rather than vice versa. On these grounds, he rejects the assumption that actions can be explained in terms of individuals' understandings, beliefs or desires. Instead, actions are the effects of what he terms 'social practices'. These practices are holistic entities or structures, the most important of them being economic practice, ideological practice and politico-legal practice. According to Althusser, individuals should not be seen as intentional actors who make their own history but as occupants of social positions that are determined by the nature and relations of the social practices in society. Thus, on Althusser's reading of Marx, within economic practice, our actions are determined by our position in the relations of production, that is, by whether we do or do not own and control the means of production. The influence of social practices upon the way in which we think is so great that that they even generate people's conception of themselves as self-conscious intentional agents.

It may be that this extremely brief explication of structuralism will serve only to confuse rather than to enlighten. Don't be too worried about the daunting nature of this theoretical position: if you can follow what Craib had to say in the above quotation, you will have grasped enough for our purposes. Basically, the reason for including the discussion here is to point out that while, apart from our examination of Durkheim and his use of sociological structuralism to explain suicide, we are not going to look at structuralism in its own terms, its importance within the corpus of sociological theory needs to be recognised. This is because it represents one of the two great poles in sociological theory, the other being the interpretative approaches discussed in Part II. While interpretative approaches assert the fundamental importance of the individual and discount social structures, structuralism denies the importance of individuals in favour of the fundamental influence of social structures.

One of the most important strands in recent sociological theorising has consisted of efforts to overcome this dualism between structure and action, and to develop models of social theory that can give due account to both. In Chapter 7, we will see how Jürgen Habermas attempts to do this through his examination of the relationship between 'lifeworld' and 'system'. Even more explicitly, Chapter 8 will address Anthony Giddens' structuration theory and Roy Bhaskar's critical realism, both of which, in different ways, seek to transcend this old argument between structuralists and action theorists.

However, this division between structure and action is not the only one that social theorists have attempted to overcome. You will remember from Chapters 3 and 4 that one of the great divisions in sociological theory lay in the differences between the ideas of Karl Marx and Max Weber. One of the most powerful attempts to synthesise the positions of these theorists can be found in critical theory. It is thus to critical theory that we now turn.

7 Critical theory and communicative action

Introduction

I hesitate to say this, but I am afraid that this chapter, more than most thus far, is rather long on the social theory and short on nursing practice. There is a reason for this. The topic that we are going to examine is not at all easy. Embedded as it is in the complex intellectual world of German philosophy, there is no quick way of explaining it. On the grounds that a rapid sweep would merely leave readers puzzled, I have opted for going through critical theory at a deliberating pace. The chapter starts by examining the roots of critical theory in classical German philosophy. It then goes on to address the ideas of the first wave of critical theorists, paying especial attention to Horkheimer, Adorno and Marcuse. I then move on to the central figure of the discussion, Jürgen Habermas, and his theory of communicative action. Following this, we get to health care issues. Two approaches are taken. First, I review critical theory critiques of medicine, and then I go on to recount my own Habermasian analysis of the adoption of communicative action in new nursing.

The roots of critical theory

The first thing that needs to be done in this chapter is to give some idea of what is actually meant by the term 'critical theory'. One way to look at it is as one of the major moments in the development of classical German philosophy, a philosophy that is in many ways distinct. Almost all critical theorists of note were (and are) German, and, unsurprisingly, their ideas are deeply embedded in that intellectual tradition. In order to map out what is meant by critical theory, I shall briefly review some ideas from three philosophers in the German tradition who had a considerable influence on the formulation of its approach.

The first application of a critical approach was made by the Enlightenment philosopher, Immanuel Kant (1724–1804), who argued that we could not simply take reason or knowledge for granted. For Kant, understanding came from a critical engagement with the conditions that make knowledge and reason possible. In other words, simply accepting the ways in which we think about things leads to superficiality; a deeper engagement with the human condition requires us to question why we think the way we do. This leads us to be critical about the assumptions that we normally make.

From his critique of knowledge, Kant (1907 [1781]) came to the conclusion that all we can ever know is the appearances of things, appearances being the result of the interaction between the outside world and human consciousness. For Kant, we could never get beyond this to really know the world outside us. Put another way, our knowledge consists of our world of experience, of 'phenomena' (this is not the first time in this chapter that we will return to the ideas of Chapter 6), which is distinct from the world of things as they actually are, which are as they are, independently of how we think about them.

This approach to human knowledge was challenged by another great German philosopher, Georg Wilhelm Friedrich Hegel (1770–1831), who maintained that Kant was incorrect in his separation of appearances from the objective world. Hegel (1977 [1807]) argued that, through self-knowledge, it was possible to uncover the basic structures of reality. Hegel contended that if we look at human history, we can see the progressive development of human self-knowledge, or the consciousness of freedom as he termed it. Through struggles and setbacks, we can see that the gradual emergence of this consciousness of freedom has provided humanity with an ever-closer approximation of the truth. For Hegel, landmarks in the progress of humanity included the emergence of Christianity (which instead of keeping its worshippers in the thrall of external gods, made it possible to worship a god in human form), the Reformation (which enhanced the freedom of individuals and debunked much of the mysticism of the medieval Church) and constitutional government (which promoted individual freedom and political rationality). Thus, for Hegel, history was a process whereby the authentic human spirit emerged from the constraints that ignorance and superstition had imposed upon it.

Hegel believed that the human spirit was the dynamo that drove history on. However, this assertion of the importance of ideas was rejected by the third German philosopher I wish to consider, Karl Marx. Instead, Marx asserted the significance of material conditions and, specifically, the social and economic relations pertaining at any given time. He argued that if we are to understand society, we need to examine the historical forms that those conditions and relations take. In contemporary society, the material conditions include advanced industrial production, and the historical form of social and economic relations involves a small group of people owning and controlling those productive forces, the rest having no control. In short, we have capitalism, which is an inherently exploitative system of human organisation. A longer discussion of Marx's social theory can be found in Chapter 3.

Critical theorists took key ideas from all three thinkers. From Kant, they accepted the need to look beneath the surface of knowledge to examine the conditions that make it possible to know. From Hegel, they took their belief in the possibility of human authenticity and freedom. From Marx, they identified the exploitative nature of capitalism. Furthermore, they argued that the ideology of capitalism (the belief system that it engenders) systematically distorts reality, in order either to conceal or to legitimate the exploitative relations that are part and parcel of the capitalist system.

To put all these ideas together, critical theory entails looking beneath the surface of knowledge and reason (Kant) in order to see how that knowledge and reason is distorted in an unequal and exploitative society (Marx) and, in doing so, to point the way to less distorted forms of knowledge and reason (Hegel).

In a way, this identification of three thinkers as the progenitors of critical theory is somewhat arbitrary. As we shall see, critical theorists are known for their wide trawls, and imaginative uses, of ideas from many sources. Indeed, one of the ways of looking at critical theory is to see it as an attempt to synthesise the radical aspects of a number of philosophical strands. Specifically, they attempted to include ideas emanating from both phenomenology and Weberian sociology in their rather loose interpretation of Hegelian Marxism. It is for this reason that I have included this chapter in Part III. I should also point out that, rather than involving a very definite and coherent programme, there is considerable variation in the ideas and approaches of critical theorists.

The Frankfurt school

Another name for the most prominent group of critical theorists is the Frankfurt school. Believe it or not, this is because they worked together in Frankfurt. More specifically, they were associated with the Institute of Social Research, which was founded in Frankfurt in 1923, was relocated in New York a decade later following Nazi persecution, and was re-established in Frankfurt in the early 1950s. The school attracted a quite exceptional group of talented people, with a wide range of interests. The group included Max Horkheimer, a philosopher and sociologist who coined the term 'critical theory'; Theodor Adorno, who, in addition to his philosophical and sociological work, was a noted musicologist; Friedrich Pollock, an economist; Erich Fromm, a psychoanalyst and social psychologist; Herbert Marcuse, a philosopher; Leo Lowenthal, a pioneer in cultural studies; and, at the edges of the group, Walter Benjamin, a literary critic.

What all these people had in common was an adherence to Marxism. However, their Marxism was coloured by the circumstances in which they found themselves. From its first formulation by Marx himself, Marxism had offered the hope of freedom and the end of exploitation. After all, capitalism, by its very nature, was sowing the seeds of its own destruction, and it was only a matter of time before the dynamics of history led to the advent of socialism. However, history had not quite gone that way. Indeed, it could almost be interpreted as running in the opposite direction. In western Europe, the 'crises of capitalism' entailed by World War I and the Great Depression had not led to a unified working class movement capable of challenging the capitalist class. Indeed, in Germany, where the critical theorists were initially based, the crises had led to the rise of Nazism and its subsequent crushing of communist opposition. On emigration to America, although life was certainly more comfortable than that under Hitler, the prognosis for working class revolution was hardly more favourable. The critical theorists confronted a self-confident capitalist society in which most of the working class seemed to accept the system. To make matters worse, in the one place where a proletarian revolution had been successfully carried out, the early promises of Bolshevik Russia were rapidly being undermined by the repressive regime of Joseph Stalin.

For the Frankfurt theorists, there was clearly something lacking in the historical approach taken by traditional Marxism. They adopted two main lines of critique. The first honed in on its scientific pretensions. The assumption that there were laws of history that were propelling humanity towards the inevitable arrival of a socialist nirvana were regarded as naïve in the face of what was actually happening in terms of historical development. For critical theorists, the downfall of capitalism was far from being an inevitability. This observation closely related to the second line of attack. Traditional Marxism was accused of being narrowly 'economistic', that is, it concentrated too much on economic relations, ignoring other important factors in the constitution of societies. Most notably, those of the Frankfurt school identified the importance of culture and ideology in the maintenance of social relations. For traditional Marxists, these areas were merely 'superstructural'; in other words, they were built on the fundamental base of material conditions and economic relations, and did not enjoy any independent status from that base. For the Frankfurt school, those forces which influenced and moulded human consciousness were of the utmost importance. After all, capitalism had suffered huge economic crises both during and after World War I, but had managed to survive, largely because the proletariat, identified by traditional Marxism as the class that would actively overthrow capitalism, had failed to do so, at least in part because many of its members had not interpreted their role in life as being part of the revolution. In other words, they had been integrated into the culture of capitalism.

The dialectic of enlightenment

As you may have noted, the critical theorists of this era were not the most optimistic bunch. This bleak outlook is graphically represented by Horkheimer and Adorno's seminal work, the *Dialectic of Enlightenment* (1978 [1947]), in which they argued that the working class revolution had failed to materialise in advanced capitalist societies, as had been predicted by traditional Marxists, because of the control that capitalism had over the consciousness of the proletariat through the development of a very powerful cultural industry. At the same time, the promise of science and reason to free individuals from mysticism and superstition had degenerated under capitalism into a tyranny of technological domination:

> the individual is wholly devalued in relation to the economic powers, which at the same time press the control of society over nature to hitherto unsuspected heights... The flood of detailed information and candy-floss entertainment simultaneously instructs and stultifies mankind.
>
> (Horkheimer and Adorno 1978: xiv–xv)

As the title of their book suggests, the target of Horkheimer and Adorno's analysis was wider than contemporary capitalism: it encompassed the entire Enlightenment project and what that project stood for. In narrow terms, the Enlightenment refers to the eighteenth-century philosophical movement which advocated the adoption of reason, systematic investigation and individual liberty, as opposed to tradition, religious revelation and monarchical rule. In wider terms, it refers to the increasing dominance of rational approaches to our understanding and control of the world. Horkheimer and Adorno argue that there are two sides to the Enlightenment. On the beneficial side, it freed humanity from a great deal of mysticism and superstition. However, the Enlightenment also contained an increasingly powerful negative aspect, and it is on this negative aspect that Horkheimer and Adorno concentrate.

The ultimate form of understanding promoted by the Enlightenment was scientific knowledge. However, as the great Elizabethan philosopher of science, Francis Bacon (1868 [1605]), recognised, the sovereignty of humanity in the world rests on its knowledge, and therefore science, as the most advanced form of knowledge, provides the instrument with which to control nature. Thus, nature is not seen as something valuable in itself but rather something to be used:

> For Horkheimer and Adorno... the domination of nature denotes a particular type of relationship between human beings and nature. Nature has meaning in so far as it has utility – in so far as it is instrumental to human purposes. Matter is *defined* as a possible object of manipulation.
>
> (Held 1980: 154)

Science, on this account, is reduced to the status of a knowledge base for technology, which is in turn used to control and manipulate. Put another way, rather than being used to understand the world as fully as possible, human rationality is reduced to the process of identifying the most efficient means with which to control the world. This is not just a matter of manipulation of the natural world outside humanity. As Held goes on to say, 'People, embodying the natural, are also potentially controllable' (1980: 154).

One-dimensional man

Scientific pretensions to understand the social world in the same manner as the natural world reached their height with the development of positivism. You may remember mention in Chapter 2 of Auguste Comte, the founding father of positivism. The ideas of Comte are examined by another of the leading critical theorists, Herbert Marcuse. Before addressing Marcuse's critical analysis of positivism, I should point out that his position was not wholly negative, in that he admitted that 'the positivist method certainly destroyed many theological and metaphysical illusions and promoted the march of free thought, especially in the natural sciences' (Marcuse 1961: 327).

Marcuse addresses Comte's assertion that the methods of the natural sciences are appropriate for the study of society. Comte makes this claim on the basis of his identification of society being constituted by events that are governed by general laws. Just as the biologist or physicist looks for general laws in nature, so the sociologist should look for general laws in society. The problem for Marcuse here is that, if we accept that the form of society equates with the form of the natural world, each being governed by iron laws, we deny the possibility of radically transforming society. For positivism:

> Social study was to be a science seeking social laws, the validity of which was to be analogous to that of physical laws. Social practice, especially the matter of changing the social system, was herewith throttled by the inexorable. Society was viewed as governed by rational laws that moved with a natural necessity.
>
> (Marcuse 1961: 343)

Thus, for Marcuse, Comte's insistence that we should look upon society as we look at nature was an inherently reactionary position, in that it assumed that the social *status quo* was as immutable as, for example, the natural law of gravity. 'Order in science and order in society merge into an indivisible whole. The ultimate goal is to justify and fortify this social order' (Marcuse 1961: 345).

The influence of phenomenology

This is not the first time in this book that we have come across criticisms of positivism. It will be remembered from Chapter 6 that Husserl attacked positivism on the grounds that it failed to recognise the active component of human consciousness. Similarly, positivism is berated by phenomenologists for its 'subject–object' dualism, whereby it regards the observer as being radically separated from the observed. For Heidegger, such a position ignores the fact that human existence and consciousness are a matter of 'being-in-the-world'.

Critical theorists were aware of their affinities to the phenomenological movement. Indeed, the debt of critical theory to phenomenology is considerable. It will be remembered that, while they were essentially Marxists, the Frankfurt school criticised traditional Marxist analyses for their concentration on economic issues to the cost of a rigorous analysis of culture and ideology. In other words, capitalism was not simply a matter of economic exploitation; it also involved an exploitative manipulation of the human consciousness. The social alienation involved in capitalism meant that 'basic dispositions towards love, friendship and community are increasingly denied and limited as their areas of expression are annexed by the commodity market' (Schoolman 1980: 37). In addition to persuading us that we are what we buy, capitalist ideology leads us to accept the day-to-day drudgery of our working lives, the mindless pap that we accept as entertainment, the unequal distribution of resources that leave many starving, to name but a few aspects of capitalism's influence on the consciousness of 'one-dimensional man', to use the words of Marcuse's (1964) famous book title.

Marcuse believed strongly in the Marxist analysis of the causes of alienation under capitalism (see Chapter 3 for a summary of that analysis). However, he also maintained that it would not be possible to overcome that alienation without the development of a critical free consciousness among those who were oppressed by capitalism. Scientific Marxism could not by itself account for how human consciousness would be able to go beyond the ways of thinking promoted by capitalism in order to be able to change it. As a result, Marcuse proposed that Marxism should be combined with the phenomenology of Martin Heidegger (Kearney 1994). Phenomenology provides us with a method of understanding lived experience and how that lived experience can transcend the constraints that are imposed on it by an alienating culture. However, phenomenology on its own was, for Marcuse, a rather hazy and idealistic philosophy that made little attempt to take account of how the material conditions in which people live influence and shape their lived experiences. This was where Marxism, with its critique of the material constraints imposed upon human existence by capitalism, came in:

> where phenomenology penetrates to the underlying existential structures of human experience, historical materialism [Marxism] grasps the material conditions of its historical configurations. In other words, if dialectical theory [Marxism] must become more concretely existential, phenomenological theory must become more concretely committed.
>
> (Kearney 1994: 207)

Thus, for Marcuse, a synthesis between Marxism and phenomenology was able to overcome the weakness of both as well as reinforcing their strengths. Marxism had the capacity to provide insight into wider social and historical forces and how those affected the condition of humanity, while phenomenology could ground those rather general insights at the level of the lived experience of individual persons. Marcuse hoped that, together, Marxism and phenomenology could develop an alternative to the *status quo* and open up the possibility of a free society in which individuals would have the opportunity fully to develop their faculties.

Habermas and communicative action

Having made our way through the difficulties of early critical theory, we have arrived at the point at which we can discuss the ideas of the great second wave critical theorist, Jürgen Habermas (1929–). Unfortunately, I have to admit that, with Habermas, things do not get any easier. If anything, he is even more eclectic in his adoption of ideas and complex in their development than the previous critical theorists whom we have been discussing. In order to keep our discussion manageable, so that we can finally get around to applying all this theory to nursing, I will limit the discussion to his use of three thinkers, all of whom we have come across before, namely Marx, Weber and Schutz.

As far as Marx is concerned, Habermas' (1972) approach is very similar to that of the earlier critical theorists. While he accepts the general thrust of the Marxist critique of capitalism, he argues that Marx gives too much primacy to material conditions and underplays the importance of ideas. On Habermas' reading of Marx, the way in which we think about things and reflect upon our situation is determined by the social and material circumstances in which we find ourselves. Part of the problem here is that Marx identifies the core attribute of humanity as the capacity to labour (see Chapter 3 for a longer discussion of this issue). Labour, and the relations in which it is carried out, is at the core of Marx's social theory. For Habermas, there is another equally important unique attribute to humanity – the ability to think and to understand – which is in turn a function of our capacity to communicate through the use of language (here we can see the influence of yet another thinker whom we discussed in Chapter 5 – George Herbert Mead):

> What raises us out of nature is the only thing whose nature we can know: language. Through its structure, autonomy and responsibility are posited for us. Our first sentence expresses unequivocally the intention of universal and unconstrained consensus.
>
> (Habermas 1972: 314)

Thus, it is both our capacity to mould our environment through labour and, more importantly for Habermas, our capacity to engage in symbolic interaction that differentiate us from other species. Human freedom is thus defined on the one hand as the ability to labour in non-alienating circumstances, and on the other as the ability to communicate with each other using rationality rather than power as the tool of persuasion.

Weber's theory of rationality

While Habermas' assertion that we need to take human consciousness fully into account in our analysis of human relations fits in well with the ideas of the earlier Frankfurt school, his assertion of the importance of rationality would appear a bit at odds with the analyses of previous critical theorists who, it will be remembered, castigated contemporary rationality for the way in which it was used to dominate and control the world. This critique of Western rationality in critical theory is a theme that was developed from the writings of Weber, and it is through his own discussion of Weber that Habermas teases out the problem of rationality.

Weber argues that there are two possible types of rational action. The first he terms 'purposive-rational action', which is:

> determined by expectations as to the behavior of objects in the environment and of other human beings; these expectations are used as 'conditions' or 'means' for the attainment of the actor's own rationally pursued and calculated ends.
>
> (Weber 1968a: 24)

Purposive-rational action simply involves working out the most efficient way of attaining a certain end. What that end happens to be is of no moral concern. In other words, purposive rationality is based on technical rather than ethical considerations. This is not the case for the second category of rational action identified by Weber, that of value-rational action, which is 'determined by a conscious belief in the value for its own sake of some ethical, aesthetic, religious or other form of behavior, independently of its prospects of success' (Weber 1968a: 24–5). In contrast to purposive rationality, value rationality concerns itself with the issue of which ends are to be valued and which means to those ends are morally justified.

It was Weber's thesis that, despite its initial foundation in the value rationality of Calvinist Protestantism, capitalism rapidly degenerated into the most oppressive form of purposive-rational action that history had seen. He sets this argument out in the conclusion of his famous study, *The Protestant Ethic and the Spirit of Capitalism* (1930 [1904–5]). In this book, Weber argues that the explanation for the rise of capitalism in the West can be found in the ideas and attitudes of Protestantism. The Protestant belief in a worldly calling, which saw practical everyday activities as being part of religious devotion, made the making of money part of the religious ethic. Moreover, anxiety over whether or not they were one of the chosen few who were predestined for Heaven meant that Protestants searched for signs of grace. One such sign was earthly success, which provided a strong motivation to prosper in business. At the same time, Protestant asceticism (adherence to the simple life) discouraged the consumption of material luxuries. As a result, instead of spending what they made, Protestant entrepreneurs reinvested their profits, thus financing the expansion of capitalism. In addition, Protestantism encouraged rational business practices, transactions being conducted in a systematic fashion and projected costs and profits being carefully assessed.

While the initial development of capitalism was the result of the deep religious ethic of reformed Protestants, its success sowed the seeds of the downfall of that ethic, in that, as time went on, the pursuit of profit in capitalism, along with the material benefits that profits brought, became ends in themselves. It is at this point that Weber sees the rise of the soulless, purposive rationality that now dominates the world. Weber's words on this issue are sufficiently chilling and eloquent to be quoted at length:

> The puritan wanted to work in a calling; we are forced to do so. For when asceticism was carried out of the monastic cells into everyday life, and began to dominate worldly morality, it did its part in building the tremendous cosmos of the modern economic order. This order is now bound to the technical and economic conditions of machine production which to-day determine the lives of all the individuals who are born into this mechanism, not only those directly concerned with economic acquisition, with irresistible force. Perhaps it will so determine them until the last ton of fossilized coal is burnt. In Baxter's [an early Protestant theologian] view the care for external goods should only lie on the shoulders of the 'saint like a light cloak, which can be thrown aside at any moment'. But fate decreed that the cloak should become an iron cage.
>
> Since asceticism undertook to remodel the world and to work out its ideals in the world, material goods have gained an increasing and finally

an inexorable power over the lives of men as at no previous period in history. To-day the spirit of religious asceticism... has escaped from the cage. But victorious capitalism, since it rests on mechanical foundations, needs its support no longer. The rosy blush of its laughing heir, the Enlightenment, seems also to be irretrievably fading... For of the last stage of this cultural development, it might well be truly said: 'Specialists without spirit, sensualists without heart; this nullity imagines that it has attained a level of civilization never before achieved'.

(Weber 1930: 181–2)

Habermas on rationality

For Weber, in its dissolution of the human soul to the level of 'pure utilitarianism', capitalism had plunged us into the 'iron cage' of purposive rationality. In large part, Habermas' project is to provide an escape route from this cage. That said, he is no doubt that the cage exists and, indeed, has become ever more constraining as capitalism has developed since the time of Weber:

In the middle decades of this century, mass education, increasing social mobility, and in short the whole process of 'modernization and development' brings with it not rationality and emancipation but rather, to Habermas's eye, a deepening *irrationality*. Late capitalism brings with it the manipulation of public opinion through the mass media, the forced articulation of social needs through large organizations, and in short, the management of politics, by 'the system'.

(Pusey 1987: 90)

According to Habermas, the twentieth century has seen the rise of what he terms 'technocratic consciousness' (1971). This entails the most severe challenge to value rationality yet seen in history. In almost all areas of life, ranging from philosophy through education to politics, the answers to problems are increasingly seen as technical rather than ethical issues. The rise of the scientific or technical expert, with the answers to any problems that may beset us, from the doctor who prescribes valium to solve one's personal unhappiness to the economist who prescribes intensive industrial growth with little concern for its environmental effects, indicates the huge expansion of technical power and the corresponding 'repression of ethics... as a category of life' (Habermas 1971: 112).

Daunting as the rise of purposive rationality in the form of technocratic conscious may be, Habermas is not despondent. As I have said, his aim is to provide a viable escape route from Weber's iron cage. He attempts to do this through the argument that Weber's portrayal of the modern world is one-sided in its assumption that value rationality has been vanquished for ever. In contrast, Habermas, while accepting the power of Weber's diagnosis, continues to hold on to the 'counterfactual' ideal of the rehabilitation of value rationality in Western societies. Habermas uses the term 'counterfactual' because, while his aspiration stands against the factual reality of the current situation, it provides the standard for a yet to be achieved, more rational social order (Pusey 1987). By reasserting the importance of value rationality, Habermas hopes to demonstrate the means by which the dehumanising effects of slavish adherence to purposive rationality can be counteracted.

The question then becomes: which values should animate a value rationality appropriate for the late twentieth century? Here we return to Habermas' assertion of the centrality of language to human nature and identity. It will be remembered that Habermas argued that human freedom should be seen in terms of the ability to communicate, persuade and be persuaded on rational grounds. Here, we have the values that animate the rationality proposed by Habermas. He uses the term 'communicative action' to describe this liberatory form of value-rational action, which is manifest in situations in which:

> the actions of the agents involved are coordinated not through egocentric calculations of success but through acts of reaching understanding. In communicative action participants are not primarily oriented to their own individual successes; they pursue their individual goals under the condition that they can harmonize their plans of action on the basis of common situation definitions. In this respect the negotiation of definitions of the situation is an essential element of the interpretative accomplishments required for communicative action.
>
> (Habermas 1984: 285–6)

The manner in which this 'negotiation of definitions' occurs is crucial. Only if negotiation is carried out without the use of power or coercion by one side or the other can it be properly regarded as rational. This sort of egalitarian interaction is termed by

Habermas the 'ideal speech situation', in which differences are rationally resolved through communication that is free from compulsion and in which the force of the better argument is the

communicative action with
...acts with an orientation to
...eech acts' (1984: 289). In
...rientated to understanding,
...success. Three forms of
...is open strategic action, in
...er to hide the fact that she
...speaker may indulge in
...her to believe that she is
...ction, while in reality she is
...ends. Third, the speaker
...ring into what Habermas
...ication'. Here, he relies on
...ample to the generation of
...nconscious repression of
...forms of strategic action
...on by purposive rationality,
...ositive value rationality on
...other.

the importance of rational communicative action. After all, if it is language that makes us human, it follows that anything that distorts free communication will also lead to a distortion of our human potentiality. Conversely, modes of interaction that promote free communication will also promote the development of our humanity: 'In so far as we master the means for the construction of the ideal speech situation, we can conceive the ideas of truth, freedom and justice' (Habermas 1970: 372).

Lifeworld and system

Before moving on to address how Habermas' ideas can be used to interrogate issues concerning health and health care, I wish to make brief mention of the latest turn in his theoretical odyssey. This is his examination of the relationship between what he calls the 'lifeworld' and the 'system' (Habermas 1987). Its importance lies in the fact that it is Habermas' most concerted attempt to overcome the division between interpretative approaches to sociology, which concentrate on individuals and their interactions, and more systems-orientated approaches that focus on large-scale social structures. On their own, Habermas regards both of these approaches as inadequate. A full understanding of the social world requires that the insights of both should be combined.

You may remember from Chapter 6 that the term 'lifeworld' was used by Alfred Schutz to denote the world constructed of taken-for-granted assumptions that form our 'intuitive environment', in which 'we, as human beings among fellow-beings, experience culture and society, take a stand with regard to their objects, are influenced by them and act upon them' (Schutz 1966: 116). Habermas accepts the significance of the importance of the lifeworld as the 'symbolic space' in which our personality and culture are not only experienced, but also sustained and reproduced (Thompson 1984). He links the notion of lifeworld to his own concerns through the observation that it is a shared, intersubjective world and thus sustained by communication. The question then becomes the manner in which our lifeworlds are constituted by communication – is this done through strategic action or through communicative action? Optimisation of our human potential comes through the positive value rationalisation of the lifeworld in the form of communicative action, which will bring to the surface for consideration previously taken-for-granted assumptions, exposing them to rational criticism and negotiation.

While the notion of the lifeworld fits in well with Habermas' theory of communicative action, he believes it can provide only a partial picture. He takes the phenomenological/*Verstehen* approach to task for concentrating too much on the internal dynamics of individuals and thus ignoring the salience of social and material conditions (echoes of Marx again):

> A *verstehende* sociology that allows society to be wholly absorbed into the lifeworld ties itself to the perspective of self-interpretation of the culture under investigation; this internal perspective screens out everything that inconspicuously affects the sociocultural lifeworld from the outside.
>
> (Habermas 1987: 148)

Habermas the 'ideal speech situation', in which differences are rationally resolved through communication that is free from compulsion and in which the force of the better argument is the only kind of force that is used.

In this manner, Habermas contrasts communicative action with 'strategic action', in which one speaker 'acts with an orientation to success and thereby instrumentalizes speech acts' (1984: 289). In other words, communicative action is orientated to understanding, while strategic action is orientated to success. Three forms of strategic action are identified. First, there is open strategic action, in which there is no attempt by the speaker to hide the fact that she has some goal in mind. Second, the speaker may indulge in conscious deception, giving the listener to believe that she is playing by the rules of communicative action, while in reality she is manipulating the situation for her own ends. Third, the speaker may be unconsciously deceptive, entering into what Habermas terms 'systematically distorted communication'. Here, he relies on psychoanalytic theory, pointing as an example to the generation of defence mechanisms as part of the unconscious repression of conflicts. The basic point is that all these forms of strategic action represent the distortion of communication by purposive rationality, while communicative action provides a positive value rationality on which to base our interactions with each other.

Considerable claims are made about the importance of rational communicative action. After all, if it is language that makes us human, it follows that anything that distorts free communication will also lead to a distortion of our human potentiality. Conversely, modes of interaction that promote free communication will also promote the development of our humanity: 'In so far as we master the means for the construction of the ideal speech situation, we can conceive the ideas of truth, freedom and justice' (Habermas 1970: 372).

Lifeworld and system

Before moving on to address how Habermas' ideas can be used to interrogate issues concerning health and health care, I wish to make brief mention of the latest turn in his theoretical odyssey. This is his examination of the relationship between what he calls the 'lifeworld' and the 'system' (Habermas 1987). Its importance lies in the fact that it is Habermas' most concerted attempt to overcome the division between interpretative approaches to sociology, which concentrate on individuals and their interactions, and more systems-orientated approaches that focus on large-scale social structures. On their own, Habermas regards both of these approaches as inadequate. A full understanding of the social world requires that the insights of both should be combined.

You may remember from Chapter 6 that the term 'lifeworld' was used by Alfred Schutz to denote the world constructed of taken-for-granted assumptions that form our 'intuitive environment', in which 'we, as human beings among fellow-beings, experience culture and society, take a stand with regard to their objects, are influenced by them and act upon them' (Schutz 1966: 116). Habermas accepts the significance of the importance of the lifeworld as the 'symbolic space' in which our personality and culture are not only experienced, but also sustained and reproduced (Thompson 1984). He links the notion of lifeworld to his own concerns through the observation that it is a shared, intersubjective world and thus sustained by communication. The question then becomes the manner in which our lifeworlds are constituted by communication – is this done through strategic action or through communicative action? Optimisation of our human potential comes through the positive value rationalisation of the lifeworld in the form of communicative action, which will bring to the surface for consideration previously taken-for-granted assumptions, exposing them to rational criticism and negotiation.

While the notion of the lifeworld fits in well with Habermas' theory of communicative action, he believes it can provide only a partial picture. He takes the phenomenological/*Verstehen* approach to task for concentrating too much on the internal dynamics of individuals and thus ignoring the salience of social and material conditions (echoes of Marx again):

A *verstehende* sociology that allows society to be wholly absorbed into the lifeworld ties itself to the perspective of self-interpretation of the culture under investigation; this internal perspective screens out everything that inconspicuously affects the sociocultural lifeworld from the outside.

(Habermas 1987: 148)

In order to take account of the outside, and 'get beyond refor-
mulations of a more or less trivial everyday knowledge'
(Habermas 1987: 148), Habermas introduces the notion of the
'system'. He argues that one of the characteristics of capitalism is
that it increasingly operates in an anonymous manner. Parts of the
capitalist system have become so complex that nobody can either
fully understand them or be held responsible for them. The
clearest instance of such a subsystem is money (McCarthy 1984).
The economic system of capitalism operates at a level that is
largely beyond the control of individuals. Unaffected by human
values, it is steered by purposive rationality.

Having escaped from the value rationality of the lifeworld,
the increasingly autonomous system threatens in turn to
'colonise' the lifeworld with purposive rationality. This is done
largely through the replacement of communicative action with
'technocratic consciousness'. In other words, rather than treating
the problems of our lifeworld as ethical dilemmas that require to
be addressed in an open and critical way, those problems are
reduced to technical issues, to be solved by those with the
requisite technical expertise. Habermas is scathing about the
soulessness of the expert:

> the life conduct of specialists is dominated by cognitive-instrumental
> attitudes toward themselves and others. Ethical obligations to one's
> calling give way to instrumental attitudes toward an occupational role
> that offers the opportunity for income and advancement, but no longer
> for ascertaining one's personal salvation or for fulfilling oneself in a
> secular sense.
>
> (Habermas 1987: 323)

Here, it might seem that we have gone full circle and are back
to the pessimism of Horkheimer and Adorno. However, this is
not quite the case, in that Habermas believes in the potential for
a value-rational lifeworld both to resist the encroachment of the
system's purposive rationality and indeed to move some way in
the other direction, so that a better balance between value and
purposive rationality might be struck. He sees practical examples
of resistance to the system in the form of pressure groups such as
ecologists, feminists and regional independence movements.
What all of these have in common is that they challenge the instrumental rationality of society and demand that the issue of values

should be reintroduced in order to guide our relations between each other and with the planet. Is it right to operate a policy of economic growth while the planet chokes? Is it right that one half of the population should be exploited on the grounds of their gender? Is it right that one's local culture should be drowned in the sea of transatlantic dross? In short, these social movements and others like them provide examples of attempts to operate 'on the basis of a rationalized lifeworld and [try] out new ways of cooperating and living together' (Habermas 1987: 394). As we shall shortly see, there may be some grounds for characterising nurses' changing relationship with clients as an example of trying new ways of co-operating and living together.

The purposive rationality of medicine

Habermas' ideas have been adopted with considerable effect in critiques of the quality of interaction between physicians and patients. For example, Eliot Mishler (1984) has critically examined the concept of patient compliance from such a perspective. Mishler argues that compliance is used to reinforce the power of medicine – only patients are non-compliant; doctors never are.

In examining interactions between patients and their physicians, Mishler distinguishes what he calls the 'voice of the lifeworld' and the 'voice of medicine'. Patients' lifeworlds consist of taken-for-granted assumptions that are grounded in the experiences of their everyday lives. In contrast, the voice of medicine entails a purposive rationality that regards events in the patients' lives as technical issues, decontextualised from particular personal or social troubles. In their interactions, physicians attempt to colonise the patients' lifeworlds. They do this by dominating interactions and controlling communication, which has the effect of undermining patients' self-understanding of the problems that they are experiencing, allowing for the imposition of the technical interpretations of the voice of medicine. Thus, the clinical practice of physicians is based on a profoundly unequal power relationship. As Mishler notes, the achievement of human care depends upon altering that relationship through empowering the voice of the patient.

The power of medical expertise

Using Mishler's theoretical construction of the physician/patient relationship as a baseline, Graham Scambler (1987) has applied a Habermasian interpretation to Graham and Oakley's (1981) analysis of the relationship between pregnant women and obstetricians. He begins by noting that the contrast between the voice of the lifeworld and the voice of medicine is well illustrated by Graham and Oakley's comparison of four areas of conflict between women's frames of reference and those of physicians. First, women generally view pregnancy and childbirth as normal processes, while physicians regard them as at least potentially pathological. Second, most women see themselves as knowledgeable about their own bodies, while physicians tend to believe that the only useful knowledge is medical knowledge and that they are the only true experts. Third, women wish to retain control over what happens, while physicians think that they have the right to make all decisions. Fourth, women often complain about the quality of communication with obstetricians: they feel pressure not to ask questions, and when they do, they are often ignored. In contrast, physicians tend to interpret questions as being symptomatic of anxiety rather than requests for information, and either do not respond or give vague answers. Scambler expands on this issue, using a transcript of interactions between a pregnant woman and a registrar, demonstrating how the physician adopts both manipulation and open strategic action in order to ensure that the reluctant woman accepts the need for induction.

The colonisation of the voice of the lifeworld is not simply a matter of the technocratic consciousness of physicians. The circumstances in which these interactions take place also tend to promote purposive rationality to the cost of communicative action. In the clinics they attended, the women usually saw a different obstetrician on each visit. Moreover, with long waiting lists, consultations were carried out on an assembly line basis. In one clinic examined, the length of time per encounter was 3.9 minutes. As a consequence, there was very little opportunity to build up the sort of rapport needed if genuine negotiation was to take place.

It can be seen how, through his use of the evidence compiled by Graham and Oakley, Scambler has demonstrated the degree to which women's lifeworlds have been colonised by the voice of purposive-rational medicine. Thus far, we have a rerun of the sort of pessimism that Weber so enjoyed, in that it would seem that technocratic consciousness has won the day. However, in line with Habermas, Scambler looks for resistance to the colonisation of the lifeworld. Here, there are signs of hope. Scambler notes the emergence of a number of user organisations, such as the Association for the Improvement of Maternity Services (AIMS) and the National Childbirth Trust (NCT), whose purpose is to articulate the wants of pregnant women and to challenge the appropriateness of high-technology, hospitalised childbirth. He argues that this development of organised resistance to the medical system can be equated with the protest movements that Habermas argued were defending the lifeworld against the encroachment of the system. Moreover, when allied to the goals of the women's movement, with its general demands for women's liberation, these groups, with their particular demands about a specific aspect of women's lives, will become an even greater force to be reckoned with.

It might be noted at this point that there is some evidence that Scambler's prognostications show some signs of fulfilment. For example, the *Changing Childbirth* report (Department of Health 1993) marked a change in government policy, towards the encouragement of choice for women in the location and manner of childbirth. While, as we shall see in the next chapter, the battle is far from won, enough has happened to warrant the hope that things are changing.

To conclude, Scambler's analysis epitomises the critical theoretical approach, in that it involves a trenchant attack upon processes antagonistic to the free development of people's humanity, while at the same time identifying avenues whereby that humanity can be rescued:

> It has been argued that system rationalization in relation to medicine... has led to a colonization of the lifeworld [of pregnant women]; that systematically distorted communication and manipulation by physicians are aspects of this process of rationalization; and that system rationalization needs to be balanced by accelerated rationalization of the lifeworld.
>
> (Scambler 1987: 190)

Nursing example: new nursing as communicative action

From the works of Mishler and Scambler, it can be seen that most Habermasian commentaries on health care have been highly critical of health care workers, specifically physicians, for their adherence to the voice of the system. As a nursing example, I wish to use a rather uncritical application of critical theory to the issue of health care, namely my own analysis of the altered relationship between nurse and patient that is entailed in the development of 'new nursing', entitled 'New nursing: the road to freedom?' (Porter 1994). In this study, I sought, through interviews with nurses, to uncover how the quality of their relationships with patients had altered as the result of the implementation of new nursing strategies such as advocacy and primary nursing.

I observed that the promotion of communicative action between patients and nurses was manifested in a number of related ways. First, the authoritarian atmosphere that used to exist on hospital wards had been undermined, and a far friendlier atmosphere than was previously the case was now promoted. This relaxation in nurse/patient relationships meant that patients now felt far more comfortable. The ending of what amounted to a culture of fear was identified by the interviewed nurses as one of the great benefits of new developments in nursing. This had in large part been achieved both by the ending of the taboo of talking with patients and by the introduction of continuity of care by means of the implementation of primary nursing.

Nor was it simply a matter of patients feeling more comfortable. The ending of the culture of fear also meant that patients now found it easier to communicate with nurses. This meant that, rather than having one-way interaction whereby the nursing expert colonised the lifeworld of the passive patient, there was now the possibility of dialogue, in which patients felt enabled to voice their own concerns. One of the benefits of this opportunity for dialogue was that patients felt prepared to ask questions and were thus in a position to find out a lot more about their illness and its treatment than they would previously have been. Thus, the increase in communication between nurses and patients led to an increase in patients' knowledge.

Patients' knowledge expectations were not restricted to wanting to know more about what was wrong with them. They also expected to know what was being done about it and why it was being done. No longer could nurses assume that the voice of the lifeworld had no right to be involved in decision-making processes. The days when the nurse could simply instruct a patient to lie on the bed and then launch into a procedure without further ado had gone. Nurses were now expected, especially by younger patients, both to explain and to justify their actions. This observation that part of the dynamic towards communicative action was as a result of the expectations of patients indicates that alterations in the nurses/patient relationship has not simply been a matter of altruistic nurses deciding that this would be a good idea. Scambler noted that the pressure groups promoting women-centred childbirth were part of a wider consumer health movement. Here we can see an example of the effects of that movement in another arena. Nevertheless, this is not to say that new nursing is the result of a defeat of nurses in the face of successful consumer pressure. The power of patients to monitor the actions of nurses has been facilitated by the willingness of many nurses to be open about their work. A number of nurses observed that their preparedness to be open with patients reduced the likelihood of patient antagonism towards them and thus improved the quality of their work experience. As one nurse put it:

> it's not that if you talk to people about what's going on, they are going to be watching like hawks to pounce on the least wee mistake. People are more likely like that when they aren't sure what's going on. It's then they are likely to be suspicious. If they think you are being straight with them, then they're straight with you. This is what I mean about treating them like people. It's better to treat people well because they'll appreciate it and treat you well as well. You can co-operate better which means you can do your job better.

> (quoted by Porter 1994: 273)

It should be noted that the developments in the relationship between nurse and patient recounted above was not simply a matter of individual nurses deciding to go with the tide of more egalitarian approaches. In one of the units where the nurses I interviewed worked, a nursing development unit, the involvement of patients in communicative action with nurses had become highly formalised. Here, nurses no longer drew up care plans on their own, deciding unilaterally what sort of care they thought patients required. Instead, care plans were the result of a process of negotiation between patient and nurse, which culminated in the signing of a 'contract' containing mutually acceptable nursing goals and actions.

Overall, from the evidence I gathered about the nature of communication between nurses and patients, I came to the conclusion that:

> new nursing aspires to and, to a degree, has achieved a transformation in the nurse–patient relationship. That relationship is changing from one of authority and subservience to one where the gap in power and status between nurse and patient is greatly diminished; where free communication rather than silent acquiescence of patients is increasingly valued by nurses.
>
> (Porter 1994: 273)

Is all in the garden quite so rosy? In all likelihood it is not. Indeed, in summing up, I was forced to admit that I could be accused of being overoptimistic, and while the aspiration may be there among nurses to reconstitute their relationship with patients along the lines of communicative action, the reality for many falls far short of that ideal. I put forward two reasons for what may have been an overly uncritical perspective. The first reason related to my methodology. I restricted my empirical investigation to interviews with nurses, and they were going to say those nice sorts of things about themselves anyway, weren't they? It would be more than likely that I would have got a far less glowing account of the nurse/patient relationship had I asked patients for their opinions. In my defence, I should point out that even those nurses who were openly unhappy about the more democratic turn in nurse/patient relationships, and who therefore had no axe to grind in favour of democracy, still admitted that it was happening, which would seem to indicate that there was something going on.

The second reason I gave was related to a weakness in Habermas' theory. This centres around the importance that Habermas places on language. The problem with this is that, despite his efforts to hold on to some of Marx's insights, some commentators have argued that there is a tendency to marginalise the effects of material conditions upon the possibilities of communicative action. As Ian Craib wryly notes, 'it sometimes seems that if we could just understand each other better, then everything would be all right' (1984: 212). It is certainly the case that there exist numerous material and structural barriers to the full implementation of new nursing, ranging from limits on health care expenditure to the continuing power of medicine, which will have to be tackled if new nursing is properly to succeed (Salvage 1990). However, I should point out in Habermas' defence that he would claim that his theory of communicative action does take due account of the salient points of Marxist materialism.

I would like to conclude this chapter by positing a third qualification to my argument, one that was not included in my original paper but which is true to the sentiments of Habermas' theory. You will remember that Habermas argues that late twentieth-century society is characterised by a struggle between the lifeworld and the system. In my paper, I concentrated almost exclusively on the advances of the value rationality of the lifeworld in the face of the disempowering purposive rationality of the system. In a way, my paper was not a disinterested examination of new nursing but a polemic about the promise that it held for the possibility of communicative action. That in itself can be seen as holding true to the project of critical theory, in that critical theorists do not see themselves as disengaged commentators but as intellectual activists whose aim is to change the world for the better through both their critique and their positing of a better alternative. However, by concentrating on the promise, I was in danger of underestimating the hold that the system still has over modes of health care interaction. Mindful of Scambler's (1987) observation that, while Habermas' ideas have been well worked out at a theoretical level, empirical work using his theories is still in its infancy, I would like to suggest that there is further work to be done in finding out just what the balance is between system and lifeworld in the specific area of nurse/patient relationships.

Recommended further reading

The Ellis Horwood/Tavistock series on key sociologists provides two extremely useful texts on this topic. First, there is Tom Bottomore's general analysis of *The Frankfurt School* (1984).

Second is Michael Pusey's specific study of *Jürgen Habermas* (1987). Another useful commentary on Habermas is provided by Thomas McCarthy (1984), which is to be found in his translator's introduction in the first volume of *The Theory of Communicative Action* but which relates to both volumes of that *opus magnum*. I have to say that McCarthy's account is fairly difficult, but it isn't half as difficult as Habermas himself. In relation to the application of Habermas to the sociology of health, Graham Scambler's (1987) chapter on the issue in his edited book *Sociological Theory and Medical Sociology* provides a superb synthesis of theory and observation.

8 Structuration theory and critical realism

Introduction

You will remember that Part II of this book consisted of an examination of approaches to sociology that regarded individuals, their understandings and their interactions as the fundamental basis of social life. Conversely, in Chapter 2, we saw how Durkheim regarded social structures as real things that governed the understandings and interactions of individuals. This structuralist approach was further elaborated in a brief discussion at the start of Part III. Both of these approaches, while coming to opposite conclusions, are concerned with the same basic problematic: how should we conceive of the relationship between social action and social structure?

One of the recent developments within social theorising has been an increasing dissatisfaction with one-sided approaches such as the ones mentioned above (see, for example, McLaughlin 1991). As a result, much effort has been expended by contemporary theorists in attempts to construct models of society that give due account to both social structure and social action. Two of the most prominent examples of this approach are discussed here. First, I will examine Anthony Giddens' theory of structuration, which sees structure and action as two sides of the same coin, each conditioning the other. As an example of how this sort of approach can illuminate issues pertaining to nursing practice, I include Mary Ellen Purkis' structurational critique of Patricia Benner.

The second approach to be considered is that of critical realism, which, in contrast to structuration theory, sees structure and action as separate, if closely linked, entities. The contrast with structuration theory will be highlighted through an exploration of the work of Margaret Archer. The philosophical foundations of critical realism, as set out by Roy Bhaskar, will also be examined. Finally, my analysis of how the ideologies of racism and professionalism influence interactions between doctors and nurses will be reviewed.

Giddens' critiques of interpretative and structural theories

Anthony Giddens (1938–) is probably the most renowned, and certainly the most cited, of contemporary sociological theorists. His output is prodigious and his areas of interest wide. He has written on the classical social theorists, on class and stratification, on modernity, on politics and on intimacy, to name only some of his concerns. However, what he is probably most famous for is his theory of structuration. The aim of this theory is build a model that can take proper account of both social actions and social structure, and thus transcend one of the intellectual battles that has dogged social theory for so long. Perhaps the best way to start an examination of structuration theory is to look at Giddens' assessment of the strengths and weaknesses of those schools of social theory which either concentrate on the interpretation of human thoughts and actions or emphasise the importance of social structures.

The positive critique of interpretative sociologies

To examine Giddens' approach to those theories which emphasise individual interpretation and action (which we called 'action theories' in the previous part), we can turn to his *New Rules of Sociological Method* (1976), which is subtitled 'A positive critique of interpretative sociologies' By 'positive', he means not positivist but sympathetic. In the *New Rules,* Giddens critically reviews the ideas of Schutz, Garfinkel and others.

As I have said, Giddens is highly sympathetic to the interpretative approach to sociology, arguing that the central tenet of his study is 'that social theory must incorporate a treatment of action as rationalized conduct ordered reflexively by human agents, and must grasp the significance of language as the practical medium whereby this is made possible' (1976: 8). In other words, we need to accept the importance of the fact that human beings do not act as automatons but think about what they do before they do it and act upon the basis of their decisions. Moreover, they also think about their actions after they have performed them, examining their consequences and considering whether or not they were appropriate or whether they should act in a different way the next time a similar situation presents itself – this is what is meant by being 'reflexive'. Giddens' assertion of the importance of language carries with it echoes of the linguistic turn in critical theory developed by Habermas (see Chapter 7). Because people act on the basis of their understandings of the situations with which they are confronted, and because that understanding is only made possible through language, which provides the basis for human thought, language can be seen as the bedrock of social action.

Giddens concurs with the basic tenet, shared by symbolic inter-actionists, phenomenologists and critical theorists, that the social world cannot be studied using the sorts of approach used to study the natural world. This is because the social world, unlike the natural world, is 'a skilled accomplishment of active human subjects' (1976: 154). In other words, in contrast to nature, which is not produced by people (although they can modify it), society is produced and reproduced by the actions of human beings. In using the term 'reproduction', Giddens includes both the maintenance and transformation of social structures.

For example, the family differs from gravity, in that gravity exists independently of human beings. In contrast, the family only exists because people decide to live together in certain social patterns. This means that there is nothing inevitable about the family. People are capable of creating alternative forms of living together – think, for example, of hippy communes or Israeli kibbutzim. The actions that produce society are neither random nor determined by outside sources: they are the result of the delib-erations of thinking social agents; this is why Giddens calls them 'skilled accomplishments'.

Thus far, it would seem that there is very little to differentiate Giddens from those theorists whom we encountered in Part II. However, differences there are. Giddens notes that interpretative social theories bear a close affinity to philosophical idealism, which assumes the primacy of ideas over material circumstances. This leads to a number of worrying tendencies. First, within interpretative sociologies, the exclusive concern with meaning pushes other aspects of human life out of the picture. Specifically, humans' practical involvement in material activity, whereby they actively transform the material conditions of their existence through labour, is lost sight of. Here we can see the influence of Marx upon Giddens' ideas.

Second, there is a tendency to seek explanations for social action exclusively in terms of the motivations of the actors, thereby neglecting the conditions in which the actor finds herself and the influence that these conditions will have over her understandings and motivations. Third, Giddens accuses interpretative theorists of a failure to examine how the social norms or expectations that influence our understandings at least partially reflect and reinforce inequalities of power in society.

For example, we might ask ourselves why a nurse would be motivated to follow a consultant on a ward round pushing the notes trolley, selecting the medical notes and pulling the curtains. It could be argued that such motivations arise from the conditions the nurse encountered in her training and continues to encounter in the structuring of ward work, which strongly encourage nursing deference to senior physicians. Moreover, we might argue that these conditions are embedded in wider patriarchal structures that pressurise women to indulge in what Hochschild (1983) calls the womanly art of status enhancement. In other words, the social norms to which the nurse is exposed reinforce gendered inequalities of power, to her cost. This is not to say that all nurses who push trolleys and pull curtains do so because they are motivated to do it. Undoubtedly, as a result of reflexive consideration of the underlying agenda, many resent what they are doing. However, this reinforces Giddens' point, in that we may do things that we are not motivated to do because we understand the constraints that we are under, which discourages us from avoiding those actions.

The positive critique of structuralism

Giddens (1979) has also made a similar positive critique of structuralism (you will remember our brief encounter with structuralism in the introduction to Part III), although it has to be said that he is far less positive about structuralism than he is about interpretative approaches. Here, he identifies a number of themes by which structuralism has made an important, if incomplete, contribution to social theory. Most of these are far too obscure to be of much interest here. However, to give a flavour of Giddens' approach to structuralism, I will make brief mention of two of his more important points.

The first point concerns structuralism's attempt 'to transcend the subject/object dualism' (Giddens 1979: 47). Here, he is referring to the problem that concerned Husserl so much about the radical division between the human observer and that which she observes (see Chapter 6). While phenomenology attempted to bring subject and object together within the realm of human experience, structuralists attempt to do so by placing human experience within the matrix of structures that govern it. Put another way, while phenomenology refutes the idea that human subjectivity and the objective world are separate things by asserting that the objective world is actively constructed by that subjectivity, structuralism refutes the idea that human subjectivity and the objective world are different things by asserting that subjectivity does not exist on its own but is the effect of structural systems. As Giddens points out, the problem with this swing in explanation is that 'little is gained if we merely replace subjectivism with some sort of objectivism' (1979: 47).

The second area in which Giddens sees structuralism as having made advances is in its efforts to 'de-centre the subject' (to use the appropriate structuralist jargon). This involves the assertion that human consciousness does not stand by itself as a self-contained and unified entity. Structuralists note that human consciousness – thinking – is mediated through language. They then apply Saussure's assertion that it is the structure of language that governs the nature of particular instances of speech rather than vice versa (once again, see the introduction to Part III). If human consciousness is constituted in and through language, it cannot claim the central importance that many previous philosophers ascribed to it. In so far as it challenges complacent notions that took consciousness as a given, as a basic component, Giddens sees the de-centring of the subject as a positive development. However, he is not prepared to go all the way with structuralists, in that he cannot accept that human consciousness is nothing more than an effect of deeper structures.

Giddens discusses a number of other areas in which he sees structuralism as providing a qualified contribution to social thought. However, in a mirror image of his critique of the interpretative sociologies, he argues that structuralism is flawed by its one-sidedness, which leads it to underestimate the significance of individual meanings and actions. He makes this argument in a number of stages. His first point involves acceptance of the structuralist point that society is not the creation of the individuals who live in it, and that, moreover, it will endure beyond the lifetimes of those individuals. However, he observes that structural analysis must include discussion of what he terms 'the mechanisms of social reproduction' (1984: 212), noting that structures only exist in so far as they are continually reproduced. The question then becomes: how are societies reproduced over time? Giddens' answer is that 'such continuity... exists only in and through the reflexively monitored activities of situated actors, having a range of intended and unintended consequences' (1984: 212). In other words, social structures can only continue to exist through the actions of individuals.

Take, for example, the way in which psychiatric care has historically been structured along institutional lines. For many decades, those institutions, which had enormous influence over the way in which the lives of those incarcerated in them were structured, were seen as the 'natural' way to deal with those labelled as mentally ill. However, through concerted action, grounded in the understandings of people who saw institutional care as inappropriate for the mentally ill, the number of individuals exposed to institutional psychiatric care is now considerably less than was the case 20 years ago. Thus, the decline of the psychiatric institution as a structuring force upon people's lives has been an intended consequence of the activities of social agents, who were not motivated to maintain this form of institutional structure. However, there have also been unintended consequences of these activities. It is hard to imagine that the reformers of the 1960s intended that the decline of repressive institutions should be accompanied by a corresponding increase in the number of homeless persons with mental illness, bereft of any form of psychiatric care. Reflexive consideration of this unintended consequence by actors with influence over mental health policy may in turn lead to the reintroduction of some form of modified institutional care for those deemed to benefit from it.

For Giddens, then, while both the interpretative and structuralist approaches have contributions to make, both are compromised by their one-sidedness:

> In interpretative sociologies, action and meaning are accorded primacy in the explication of human conduct; structural concepts are not notably prominent, and there is not much talk of constraint. For functionalism and structuralism, however, structure... has primacy over action, and the constraining qualities of structure are strongly accentuated.
>
> (Giddens 1984: 2)

In their attempts to create a linkage between subject and object, both interpretative sociologies and structuralism make the mistake of trying to dissolve one side of this divide into the other. Thus, interpretative sociologists dissolve structure into meaning, while structuralists attempt to dissolve meaning into structure. Giddens' solution is to see meaningful action and social structure as a 'duality'. By this he means that rather than seeing them in terms of dualism (as two separate things), or as totally one or the other (as the above approaches attempt to do), they should be seen as two sides of the one coin. This assertion lies at the core of his theory of structuration.

Structuration theory

Like Habermas in the previous chapter, Giddens, for all his sophistication, is hardly a master of the succinct. His discussions of structuration theory tend to be drowned in esoteric elaboration of secondary issues. As a result, it is difficult to get to the core of what he is on about. Probably one of the clearest definitions that he has given came in one of the first outings of the concept in the *New Rules*:

> To enquire into the structuration of social practices is to seek to explain how it comes about that structures are constituted through action, and reciprocally how action is constituted structurally.
>
> (Giddens 1976: 161)

As far as structures are concerned, Giddens argues that they do not exist independently of human action: it is human action that brings them into being. Indeed, he goes so far as speaking of structures having only a 'virtual existence' that only comes into full being when they are 'instantiated' by social action (1982: 9). What he means here is that structures only become reality when certain actions bring them to 'life'. Before attempting to explain this further, let me continue with Giddens' description of structures. He points out that much of the literature on structures is rather vague – it is rarely explicitly stated what exactly a social structure is. When structure is explicated, the picture drawn is often a very mechanical one whereby social structures are deemed analogous to natural laws. In contrast, Giddens has a very clear view of what he means when he uses the term, one which sits at a considerable distance from the traditional view of structures as mechanical laws. Structures are for him the rules and resources upon which social agents draw when acting.

Perhaps the best way of looking at the issues introduced here is through metaphor. Take the game of chess, which is governed by a set of rules. When we are neither playing nor thinking about chess, those rules, while they still exist, do not have any effect upon our lives. In other words, they have a 'virtual existence'. It is not until we decide to play a game of chess, and in doing so start to apply those rules to our conduct, that they take on a fuller reality. It is only in instances of the game being played that the rules of the game affect our actions, in that we draw upon those rules in order to engage in the activity of chess in a manner that we find mutually comprehensible with our opponent; put back into Giddens' jargon, virtual rules are instantiated through social action. Similarly with resources, we may have a bank statement to say that we have £10,000 in our savings account (I realise that this is a rather far-fetched example), but while it sits there, it has only a virtual reality as far as we are concerned. It is not until we decide to act and buy that long-awaited cruise that our actions instantiate that resource and turn it into something real.

Here, you might object that there is nothing virtual about money in the bank – it is something that is really there. Giddens notes this point but argues that material (or, in his terms, 'allocative') resources, such as land or money, only actually become resources when they are put to some use. A plot of land that is left aside to be taken over by weeds is only potentially a resource. It is only when someone comes along and ploughs, fertilises and plants potatoes on it that it becomes a resource proper.

Moreover, as well as allocative resources, Giddens identifies another class of resource, which he terms 'authoritative resources'. These involve the capacity to make fellow humans our resources by getting them to do what we wish them to do. Here, we might go back to the trolley-pushing nurse and the non-trolley-pushing consultant mentioned earlier. The actions of these two social agents on a ward round, the nurse acting in a subservient fashion and the physician in a superior one, are an example of the utilisation of the authoritative resources that structure health care occupations in favour of medicine. Without actions such as these, which practically display the occupational subordination of nursing, the authoritative resources of medicine would remain in virtual state.

For Giddens, the ability to utilise authoritative resources provides the basis of social power. However, he is wary of regarding the exercise of power as a zero sum game, in which one side has all the power and the other none. Instead, he conceives of power in a more positive light as 'the capability of the individual to "make a difference" to a pre-existing state of affairs or course of events' (1984: 14). Thus, with the exception of those who are profoundly physically or mentally disabled (that is, totally paralysed and aphasic or comatose), all of us, through our actions, have the capacity to deploy a range of causal powers. This means that:

> we should not conceive of structures of domination built in to social institutions as in some way grinding out 'docile bodies' who behave like automata... Power within social systems... presumes regularized relations of autonomy and dependence between actors or collectivities in contexts of social interaction. But all forms of dependence offer some resources whereby those who are subordinate can influence the activities of their superiors.
>
> (Giddens 1984: 16)

Thus, to return yet again to the trolley, the nurse is not simply a robot programmed to push it along behind a retinue of medics. She also has resources that she can utilise in such a situation. She could, for example, arrange for her colleagues to keep calling her away from the round in the hope that the exasperated consultant will eventually instruct one of the junior medical staff to take over. Even more brazenly, she could openly point out that she regards the practice as degrading and that, as a highly trained professional, she feels that her skills could be better used on less mundane tasks. Here, the structural resources that nursing has increasingly gained through its claim to professionalism would be used as a balance to the resources historically enjoyed by medicine. Whether or not it would work is, of course, another matter.

Essentially, what Giddens is saying is that is a mistake to conceptualise social structures as real things out there determining our lives. Social structures are only brought into existence by our actions. In other words, structures are produced and reproduced by action. Moreover, Giddens argues that only if these rules and resources are utilised over periods of time and in different circumstances can they be properly regarded as structural. As he puts it himself, 'The structural properties of social systems exist only in so far as forms of social conduct are reproduced chronically across time and space' (1984: xxi). Finally, Giddens argues that structures should not be seen in a wholly negative manner, constraining individual actions. As well as involving constraint, structures entail enablement: they allow us do things in certain ways, as well as discouraging us from doing other things.

While structures may be instantiated by action, they in turn regulate social action. Human beings are not free to live their lives and act in any old way they choose. The rules and resources of social structures regulate the possibilities of social action, providing a limited number of options for social actors. Thus, if one does decide to have a game of chess, one accepts that one should act according to certain rules. Although in social life, rules are often not as solid and unbending as they are in chess and can often be bent to suit one's aims, or even changed over time, they still provide limits to the possible actions that a person can take in any given situation.

Thus, we can see how the relationship between structure and action is circular (or, in Giddens' jargon, 'recursive'). This circle involves structures providing the possibilities and constraints within which action takes place, while action in turn produces or reproduces those structures:

> The constitution of agents and structures are not two independently given sets of phenomena, a dualism, but represent a duality. According to the notion of the duality of structure, the structural properties of

> social systems are both medium and outcome of the practices they recursively organize.
>
> (Giddens 1984: 25)

To sum up, structuration theory can be seen as Giddens' attempt to put flesh on the bones of Marx's famous dictum that people make their own history but not under conditions of their own choosing. To put too much emphasis on either the people or the conditions is to leave out important aspects of the social world. An adequate explanation must give due acknowledgement to the importance of both and to the relationship between them.

Nursing example: the intrusion of the social

As yet, there are few examples of the use of structuration theory in interrogating issues relating to nursing practice. One exception, however, is Mary Ellen Purkis' 'Entering the field: intrusions of the social and its exclusion from studies of nursing practice' (1994). Using insights from a number of philosophers and social theorists, but centring her critique around the theory of structuration, Purkis argues that there is a tendency in accounts of nursing practice to exclude recognition of the importance of social dynamics within that practice:

> Within a practice based discipline such as nursing, work is accomplished between social actors. Entering the literature, however, to discover the 'how' of practice, it is common to find prescriptions for improved communication skills and alternative definitions of nursing concepts. Only marginal attention is given to how practices such as health promotion are accomplished. This marginality arises... from the exclusion of 'the social'.
>
> (Purkis 1994: 315–16)

In contrast to this tendency to exclude the social, the aim of Purkis' paper is to 'render a description of practice which reorientates "the social", returning it to its central, *constituting* position in discussions about nursing practice' (1994: 317).

In order to demonstrate the problems that arise when commentators exclude the social from their accounts and explanations of nursing practice, Purkis provides close readings of two influential texts. Here, I will concentrate on her deconstruction of Patricia Benner's seminal analysis of the development of nursing expertise, *From Novice to Expert* (1984). Benner's study seeks to demonstrate how, with the gaining of experience, the clinical nurse progresses through various levels of practice. The first stage is that of novice, in which the nurse's behaviour is rule-governed. In other words, the novice performs her work with a high degree of dependency upon the formal knowledge and procedures: she goes by the book and does not have the confidence to rely on her own judgements. At the other end of the spectrum is the expert, whose behaviour reflects an intuitive grasp of clinical situations. This intuitive knowledge is gained through nurses learning from critical incidents, which stand out because they change the nurses' perception, leading them to view future clinical situations differently. This stock of intuitive knowledge increases over time, giving the expert nurse the confidence to rely on her own judgements.

Purkis' line of critical departure starts with the observation that Benner's construction of knowledge is one of 'naïve realism', which assumes that knowledge and language can provide a true and accurate picture of the world as it really is. In contrast, Purkis argues that 'language comes to be constituted by the nurse through interaction with others' (1994: 326). Purkis then links the issue of naïve realism with the problem of the exclusion of the social and in particular with what she sees in Benner as a blindness to the issue of how nurses construct their knowledge within the matrix of power relations:

> rather than recognizing patterns of patient behaviour, based on some fundamental knowledge, some accumulation of knowledge, the nurses, through language, constitute 'patterns'. This constitution is taken by Benner to imply the demonstration of 'expertise' by nurses. However, Benner's perspective fails to recognize the constituting nature of language. This naïve view does not question the effect of power inherent in language on the constitution of knowledge.
>
> (1994: 328)

The relationship between power, language and knowledge is crucial. Here we might remember Giddens' (1976) argument that structuration theory involves the acceptance of the significance of language as the practical medium whereby the social conduct of human agents is made possible. Through the medium of language,

agents use knowledge to organise and co-ordinate their social
actions, including power relations.

In order to demonstrate what she sees as the naïveté of Benner's
approach to knowledge, Purkis examines a selection of transcripts
of interviews with nurses used by Benner to demonstrate different
levels of knowledge. One transcript in relation to the expert nurse
relates to an intervention that a nurse made in a patient care
situation. The nurse observed a medical student and another nurse
attending to a patient. Feeling that her colleague was in considerable need of help, she entered the room:

> I had a sense of what was going on and I looked at the patient and there
> were two things that I noticed right off: One was that her abdomen was
> very large and very firm and the other that her knees were mottled. I said,
> 'she has a dead bowel'. And they said, 'She doesn't have a dead bowel'.
> And I said 'She has a dead bowel'. All right, trying to back off a little bit,
> I asked 'Would we consider that maybe she has an ischemic bowel?'
>
> (Benner *et al*. 1992: 25).

In her acceptance that this transcript provides evidence of the
successful application of intuitive knowledge, Benner takes this
account at face value as a reflection of the reality of the situation
(naïve realism again). In contrast, Purkis, rather than accepting
accounts such as the one above as being representative of an
unquestioned reality, argues that they provide evidence of how
nurses use language to constitute their work and the social
relations that such work involves. Specifically, she sees in these
accounts the use of what she terms 'discursive strategies' that are
used to prop up existing power relations. In the terminology of
structuration theory, nurses' interpretations of their actions are
used to instantiate the rules and resources that pertain in the social
world of health care work. In other words, Purkis sees these
accounts of instances whereby structures are constituted through
action, that being one side of the duality of structure. As she
observes, the social world of health care involves a hierarchy that
positions nurses between doctors and patients. However, she goes
on to point out that nurses draw on this structural feature of their
work to give meaning to their work experiences. Thus, we see
evidence of the other side of the duality of structure in that the
actions of nurses and their understanding of those actions are
constituted structurally.

Thus, Purkis reads the expert nurse's account as being constructed as a oppositional tale, which both reflects and reproduces her structural position within the hierarchy. The nurse sees herself as able to interpret symptoms accurately, but as not able to have her interpretation legitimated by the other actors in the encounter. Her reason for entering the situation on the grounds that her colleague was in 'desperate need for help' (Benner *et al.* 1992: 25) represents an implicit acknowledgement that, through the application of her knowledge, she could alter the social dynamics of the encounter:

> The statement made by the expert nurse to the nurse and the medical student was not only conveying meaning in terms of signification (Giddens 1984: 31). The message, encoded within an organizational frame of reference, results in an intertwining of meaning with normative elements (moral order) and power. The example is one of a structurated process.
>
> (Purkis 1994: 331)

However, when her intervention is not accorded legitimacy, the nurse is forced to back off, thus maintaining instead of transforming the structures of power existing between physicians and nurses.

In summary, Purkis' point is that nursing actions are inevitably social actions. Therefore, accounts of nursing actions, if they are to be adequate, must include a recognition of the social. She frames her theoretical interpretation of those actions within structuration theory, arguing that nursing actions are both constituted by and in turn constitute the structural rules and resources that pertain in health care settings.

Archer's critique of structuration theory

While Giddens' theory of structuration theory has had an enormous influence upon recent social science, it has not been without its critics. Prominent among these is Margaret Archer. The first thing to note here is that Archer (1995) agrees with Giddens that structures should not simply be seen as constraining action: they can also enable action. In other words, structures do not simply stop us doing things, but also allow us to do certain things. Archer is also at one with Giddens' analysis of both structuralist and interpretative approaches, accepting that what she calls the 'downwards conflation' of structuralism, in which agency is seen as an effect of structure, and the 'upwards conflation' of interpretivism, which sees structures as merely the aggregates of individual actions, are both erroneously one-sided. However, she goes on to argue that Giddens' attempt to escape from this one-sidedness has not been entirely successful.

Structuration theory is described by Archer as an example of 'central conflation'. By this she means that, while Giddens rejects attempts to get away from regarding structure and agency as two different entities through the reduction of one into the other, he nevertheless wishes to hold on to the idea that structure and agency are fundamentally inseparable. As Craib observes:

> instead of separate and opposing things in the world or as mutually exclusive ways of thinking about the world, they [structure and action] are simply two sides of the same coin. If we look at social practices in one way, we can see actors and actions; if we look at them another way we can see structures.

> (1992: 3–4)

In contrast, realists such as Archer ascribe to structures and actions a separate reality of their own. Archer is unhappy with the conflation of structure and action on a number of grounds. Here I will address just one – time. The choice is ironic, in that one of Giddens' claims is that previous social theory did not take the issue of time seriously enough and that 'the conception of structuration introduces temporality as integral to social theory' (Giddens 1979: 198).

Archer observes that by giving structures only a virtual reality, Giddens condemns them to a limbo outside time. It is only when they are instantiated through social actions that they come into being. In other words, it as at the same moment in time – at the same instance – that action and structure exist. Thus, one of the effects of Giddens' definition of structure and action in terms of one another is that this 'mutual constitution ultimately implies temporal conjunction between the two elements' (Archer 1995: 87). Because it conceives of structures being conjured up at the same moment as the actions they condition, 'structuration theory cannot recognize that structure and agency work on different time intervals' (1995: 89).

In contrast, Archer's realist approach asserts that structure and agency operate over different time periods. Archer accepts Giddens' point that structures cannot exist independently of social actions but asks 'whose actions?' (1995: 72). Her answer is based on Auguste Comte's aphorism that the majority of actors are the dead. The social structures that affect our lives have not been conjured up by our own instantiation of them, but rather they are the result of the actions of those who came before us in time. Think for example of the National Health Service, which structures the form and content of health care delivery in Britain. While this health care structure is the product of human actions, it is a product of actions performed before, during and immediately after World War II. Nye Bevan is long dead, yet the fruits of his labour still condition the way in which health care is structured (albeit in a modified fashion). In short, because they are the result of human actions in the past, social structures pre-date contemporary actions. Archer describes this as the stage of 'structural conditioning'.

The next stage is that of 'social interaction'. Archer argues that contemporary actions may either reproduce or transform those structures inherited from the past. Once again, transformation, when it does occur, does not happen instantaneously but takes time. There are two main reasons for this. First, not everyone in society acts in the same way. Often, there are those whose vested interests lie in the *status quo* and others with vested interests in change. Depending on the success of the former group's actions, the change desired by the latter group may be prevented or its pace slowed. Second, the structural conditions pertaining during the period of social interaction will often place limitations on the speed with which that interaction can induce change.

Think, for example, about the debate over where to be born. Supporters of home birth were faced with a health care structure ensuring that almost all children were born in hospital. They were also faced with an extremely powerful group, namely obstetricians, who wished to maintain that structure as it was. It took many years of concerted pressure before the government was finally persuaded that mothers should be given a real choice about where they wished to give birth. Even at this point, obstetricians have been very successful in slowing the momentum of a move towards home birth. For example, the Department of Health

(1993) has asked that providers of maternity care 'review their current organisation and practices to ensure that real choice about the place of birth is available'. The response to this request from the obstetric establishment has been the drawing up of long, detailed lists of selection or risk assessment criteria. The application of these ensures that birth outside obstetric units is restricted to those women deemed very unlikely to develop complications during pregnancy or labour (even though there appears to be little scientific evidence that these criteria actually predict this accurately) and those women who are prepared to exert their choice in spite of an adverse risk assessment (Campbell and Porter 1997). In this way, the medical obstetric élite has been able to slow down the pace of structural change.

Even if it were the case that there was no opposition to this development, there would still be a considerable lapse between the policy decision to allow choice of childbirth location and the development of structures to facilitate such choice. To take but one facet, because of the way in which maternity care is currently structured, most midwives have only had experience of hospital deliveries. To take on the responsibilities of assisting birth on their own in a private house would therefore require them to be 'reskilled' to enable them to cope with the new demands. As there are only a few midwives with such skills, it follows that there are few to teach such skills and, in turn, that they will be able to teach only a relatively small number of their colleagues. While in time there would be a snowballing of the number of midwives with the requisite skills, as the newly trained added to the numbers capable of teaching, the process would be far from instantaneous. Thus, we can see the time lapse between the commencement of actions designed to change structures and actual change in the structures themselves.

We now come to the last stage of the temporal process, which Archer calls 'structural elaboration'. Assuming that the aim of a particular type of action is to transform a social structure, it will, if it is successful, produce new structural properties, which will in turn provide the conditions for future actions. New social possibilities (or constraints) are gradually opened up as structural forms respond to the effects of social action, although the structures that emerge will usually not be exactly as those actors for change intended them to be. To stay with the issue of childbirth, if the actions of those currently pressing for a choice in place of birth are successful, the consequences of such a move might well extend far beyond the alteration of location. Assuming that large numbers of women decided that they wished to give birth at home with only a midwife in attendance, this would result in a significant reduction of obstetric involvement in childbirth. Given that obstetrics is a male-dominated occupation, while midwifery is female-dominated, such a move would entail women (both mothers and midwives) retaking control over an important area of women's health. Thus, the new structures would be elaborated in a fashion that involved increased enablements and fewer constraints over women's lives.

On a less optimistic note, and thinking back to what happened with the move of mental health care to the community, it might be the case that the government will use the rise of home births as a cheap alternative, radically cutting the expenditure on maternity services. This would be an unintended consequence of the actions of reformers.

Whatever the outcome, the structural elaborations that emerge would then face actors in the future as the structural conditioning for their own social interaction, and so the cycle begins again.

Bhaskar and critical realism

Archer's position can be regarded as the sociological application of a philosophical stance known as critical realism, which has been primarily developed by the British philosopher Roy Bhaskar (1944–). Bhaskar's use of the word 'realism' comes from the fact that he asserts (in contrast to idealism) that there *is* a reality out there that is independent of our observations or thoughts about it. Put another way, in common with other realist philosophies, critical realism recognises that knowledge in general, and science in particular, are *about* something – that there are objects of knowledge that exist independently of that knowledge. However, critical realism goes further than this. It asserts that reality is not confined to surface events or objects. Three levels of reality are posited: first, the empirical, which comprises experienced events; second, the actual, which consists of all events, whether experienced or not; and finally, the causal, which consists of those structural mechanisms that generate events. Despite the fact that they are not the objects of direct experience, these mechanisms are regarded as real. This is because they satisfy the causal criterion for reality: they are real because they cause events to occur (Bhaskar 1978). It is the first and third levels of reality that are of most importance for our discussion.

Take, for example, the arrangement of iron filings into patterns using a magnet. The first and most obvious level of reality here is the empirical level, which consists of those instances in which we see filings move into patterns. However, if we only accepted this level of reality, we could not explain why the filings go into the patterns that they do. In order to do this, we must also accept the reality of magnetism, which structures the movement and arrangement of those filings. Of course, we can never see or feel magnetism; we can only see or feel its effects – the movement of the filings. However, the fact that it can cause these effects is proof of its reality.

It should be noted that critical realism is not a hard determinist philosophy; it does not assert that the influence of structures are so great that if they are involved in an event, they will cause things to happen in a definite way. On the contrary, critical realism argues that because structural mechanisms cause events to occur in 'open' systems, in which more than one mechanism is operating at one time, and in which different mechanisms may promote contradictory effects, the operation of a particular mechanism cannot be identified by the constant conjunction of events. This term 'constant conjunction' comes from the Scottish philosopher, David Hume (1969 [1739–40]), who argued that the way in which we come to accept the existence of laws is through experiencing one event occurring after another over and over again. Thus, for Hume, it is through the experience that every time we drop something, it invariably falls to the ground (there being a constant conjunction between dropping and falling) that we come to the conclusion that there must be a law of gravity. Rather than accepting this notion, Bhaskar argues that structural mechanisms should be regarded as tendencies. Thus, he states that 'in citing a law one is referring to the... activity of a mechanism... not making a claim about the actual outcome (which will in general be co-determined by the activity of other mechanisms)' (Bhaskar 1989a: 9–10).

Take tuberculosis, for example. A determinist might state that infection by the tubercle bacillus will cause the disease, but this is not actually the case. It is perfectly possible to be infected yet never show signs of tuberculosis. In addition to infection, what is also required is an internal environment that will allow the disease to flourish. If that internal environment is well nourished, the chances of the bacillus taking hold are reduced because the body's capacity to resist is increased. Thus, the relationship between the tubercle bacillus and the human body takes place in an open system; it is not simply a closed matter of infection invariably causing disease but one of the possibility of infection causing disease if other, supportive causal mechanisms are present. Other pertinent structural mechanisms include the socio-economic system in which the infected person lives and the person's position within that system, which will in turn condition the person's ability to enjoy a nutritious diet. It is no coincidence, for example, that tuberculosis remains endemic among the poor of developing countries, while it is relatively rare in more affluent societies.

Critical realism is not just applied to the natural world; a similar analysis is made of the social world. Bhaskar (1989a) argues that people's actions cannot be explained simply in terms of their individual needs or desires (although he does not wish to deny the importance of those needs and desires). People's actions are not random; their behaviour also has patterns. Therefore, an adequate explanation of human action needs to include identification of the structures that influence those patterns. The word 'influence' is significant. Bhaskar does not seek to portray human beings as automatons who simply respond automatically to the dictates of social structures. Society is an open system, in which there are many structures operating simultaneously, some reinforcing and some contradicting each other. Add to this the psychological structures that we each possess, and firm prediction of the actions of specific individuals becomes impossible; the aim of the social scientist is to identify the tendencies generated by structures.

While there are similarities, social structures cannot be unproblematically equated with natural structures. The most important difference between them is that social structures are not independent of the individuals whose lives they influence; rather, they are maintained or transformed by the actions of individuals. Thus, the relationship between structure and action is a two-way process. Here we return to the concerns of Giddens. However, while this statement might appear to be consonant with structuration theory's notion of duality, both Bhaskar and Archer differ from Giddens in that they see social structures as more than the rules and resources that are instantiated through social action.

For critical realism, while structure and action are closely connected, they are different things. Thus critical realism reasserts the dualism that structuration theory seeks to deny. What then gives structures a reality over and above their instantiation in social interactions? Here we return to the ideas of Durkheim and his notion of emergent strata that was outlined in Chapter 2. This view asserts that reality is constituted by a number of layers, each layer emerging from the interrelationship of the elements of a more basic level. While the structural level of society emerges from social interaction, it has powers and properties that are 'relatively autonomous' from that action. In turn, those powers and properties exert independent influence upon social action in their own right. To use Archer's (1995) terms, structural conditioning of social interaction, while it is the product of previous social interaction, nevertheless confronts current social actors as something that is already there and which influences their options for action in ways that are not completely within their control.

Bhaskar (1989b) does not see social science as a value-free exercise. The work of the scientist is to identify patterns of social behaviour and ask what social structures must be in existence in order for those patterns to occur, and then to question empirically whether the hypotheses formulated can adequately explain the patterned activities observed. This is not just an academic exercise. Exposure of social structures, and the constraints and enablements that they impose upon our freedom to act in our own interests, provides us with knowledge that can be used in attempts to improve the structural organisation of society (hence the inclusion of the adjective 'critical' in the description of his philosophy). Here, we can see a close affinity with Marxism, which concentrated on the enablements and constraints that result from economic structures such as capitalism and communism. However, critical realism has the benefit of avoiding the dangers of 'economism' (reducing everything to the economic sphere) to which Marxism has sometimes fallen victim, in that it allows us to take account of other social structures, such as patriarchy and racism. The effects of the latter are the subject of our nursing example.

Nursing example: racism and professionalism

After my self-promotion in the previous chapter's nursing example, I am somewhat loath to do the same thing again. My justification for doing so is that few others have, as yet, utilised critical realism to promote the understanding of nursing. The paper that I will discuss here is entitled 'Critical realist ethnography: the case of racism and professionalism in a medical setting' (Porter 1993).

This paper used ethnographic data pertaining to interactions between nurses and doctors in an intensive care unit to test two hypotheses about the relationship between structures and actions. The first hypothesis was that structural racism would to some degree inform relationships between white health workers and those belonging to 'racialised' groups. The second was that the occupational structuring of health care work would affect the way in which racism was expressed.

My paper took as its starting point a study by David Hughes (1988) of nurse/doctor relations in an accident and emergency department. Hughes noted that nurses were far less deferent in their interactions with doctors who hailed from the Asian sub-continent than they were with white doctors; on occasion, they directed them to perform specific tasks, reprimanded them for their behaviour and openly criticised their professional competence. In contrast, my own research did not reveal these types of behaviour by nurses towards Asian doctors. There was clearly something significant about this discrepancy that would need to be explained if an understanding of the nature of racism in this particular context was to be achieved.

The first explanation I considered was that racism, while present in Britain, was absent in Ireland, where my research took place. However, this rather naïvely optimistic approach could not stand up in face of the evidence that when nurses were on their own, they were prepared on occasion to express their (bad) opinions of their Asian and African medical colleagues in racist terms. Moreover, there were some subtle hints in open interactions, in that nurses were noticeably cooler and more formal in their interactions with these physicians, and the physicians in turn made efforts to demonstrate that they possessed superior occupational power and health care knowledge.

The question then became: why were the nurses in the accident and emergency department prepared to voice their disdain openly, while the nurses in the intensive care unit were prepared to voice it only in private? Another possibility was that, as recent immigrants, the doctors in accident and emergency were not familiar with the culture in which they were living and working, whereas the intensive care physicians were. This lack of cultural awareness might then be linked to levels of competence to perform the tasks required of them, in order to explain why nurses felt the need to intervene. This, indeed, was how the nurses in the accident and emergency department saw things. The problem with this explanation is that, by simply treating the loss of deference as a result of a lack of physicians' competence, racism is excised from the equation altogether. We have already noted how nurses in my study expressed racist attitudes in private; we might also note the considerable evidence indicating that second- and third-generation black British people, who could hardly be described as being unfamiliar with British culture, continue to experience racism (Brown 1984).

The third explanation that I posited was framed in terms of critical realism. Noting that nurses and doctors work in a open social system, I argued that racism was not the only structure of influence upon the social interactions that occurred between white nurses and Asian and African physicians. At this point, I turned to the issue of professionalism.

I framed my analysis here in terms of Talcott Parsons' (1951) classification according to pattern variables, which were discussed in Chapter 2. This choice may seem odd, given Celia Davies' (1995) turning of these patterns on their head in her treatment of gender issues in relation to professionalism (see again Chapter 2). However, what I was arguing here was that while Parsons may not have provided an adequate analysis of professional characteristics, it was largely the case that professionals themselves (including nurses) had accepted that their occupations were characterised by the variables he describes. In other words, Parsons' typology fits in well with the self-image of professionals. Four of these variables, linked by their emphasis on the importance of rationality, are of direct relevance to the issue of racism. Affective neutrality assumes that judgements should be made on rational grounds rather than on (racist) feelings about someone. Universalism means taking an objective stance that is not influenced by irrelevant characteristics of the person with whom you are dealing. Achievement orientation entails regarding physicians as having attained their occupational status through ability, independent of ascriptive qualities such as 'race'. The final variable is role specificity, which allows physicians to be judged only on their skills as physicians rather than on factors not pertinent to the job.

Accepting that professional ideology, which is based on the sorts of notion expounded by Parsons, structures both physicians' and nurses' interpretations of what is and what is not acceptable behaviour, we can begin to see how this ideology might constrain the possibility of open racism. Given that such importance is attached to the pattern variables above:

> Naked racism, being irrational, ascriptive, particularistic, diffuse and affective, is therefore not justifiable as an open form of social interaction between nurses and doctors.
>
> (Porter 1993: 605)

However, this is where the issue of competence came in, in that it provided the perfect excuse for nurses to act in a racist fashion while still paying lip-service to the requirements of professional conduct:

> To be acceptable in this social milieu, racism needs to be cloaked in a 'rational' veneer. This is what is happening when differential competence is married to 'race'. Criticism on the grounds of competence can be portrayed as rational, affectively neutral, universalistic, achievement oriented and specific to the skills of medicine. Yet, the racism is still there. From such a perspective, criticisms of immigrant doctors' competence can be seen as the vehicle through which racism is expressed.
>
> (Porter 1993: 605)

However, in circumstances in which black physicians are cultur-ally literate, as they were in the intensive care unit, an important avenue for racism is cut off. This does not mean that racism ceases to exist but merely that the opportunities for its articulation are limited – it is submerged in the public arena but continues to find expression in private.

From this examination of the structural relationship between racism and professionalism, we can see the complexities of open social systems. While structural racism existed in both settings, its expression was modified by professional ideology. Rather than determining that white nurses would be openly racist, it generated a tendency that encouraged racism but was submerged where another, countervailing tendency (namely professional ideology) came into play.

In the actions of the Asian and African physicians in the intensive care unit, which involved using their occupational advantages, such as formal authority and clinical knowledge, to minimise the disempowering effects of racism, we can also see how agency seeks to transform social structures.

Conclusion

We have seen how there are fundamental differences between structuration theory and critical realism. However, whatever their respective strengths and weaknesses, both have the merit of taking a wider approach to the problem of structure and action than was often the case with earlier social theories. Both sought to build upon previous insights, to synthesise those insights and thus to improve upon them. In this way, they can be seen as an extension of traditional social theory. In contrast, others have come to the point at which they have decided to give up on social theory as it has been traditionally constituted, on the grounds that it contains irredeemable flaws. These attempts to break away into new territories can be found in postmodernism and some forms of feminism. It is to these that we turn in Part IV.

Recommended further reading

A good critical introduction to Anthony Giddens can be found in the eponymous book by Ian Craib (1992). For detailed discussion of various aspects of structuration theory, see Bryant and Jary's edited volume *Giddens' Theory of Structuration: A Critical Appreciation* (1991). As I have already said, Giddens' own writing tends to be rather dense, but it is nothing compared with the linguistic jungle that confronts one on opening the pages of a book by Roy Bhaskar. Going directly to Bhaskar is not for the faint-hearted. Fortunately, Andrew Collier has provided us with an accessible introduction in *Critical Realism: An Introduction to Roy Bhaskar's Philosophy* (1994).

PART IV

Taking it all apart

In the previous section, we examined attempts to overcome the divisions that have dogged social theory since its inception. In large part, critical theory, structuration theory and critical realism can be seen as extensions of classical social theory. Certainly, both critical theory and critical realism, despite the former's distrust of the way in which Enlightenment values have actually played out, remain within the Enlightenment tradition, in that they involve the rational interpretation of evidence to criticise existing conditions and thus to point to a better way forward. Despite the pessimism of critical theory, there remains a hope in the possibility of progress based on rationality, even if that rationality is of a form different from that of the purposive rationality that has dominated Western life over recent centuries.

Others are not so sanguine about this route to progress; these will be the subject matter of Part IV. The first approach to be examined is that of feminisms, in particular cultural and standpoint feminisms. Both of these involve a rejection of the traditional approaches of rationality in general and social theory in particular, which they see as entailing male-centred assumptions. Indeed, one of feminisms' criticisms of social theory is that for a long time it assumed that women simply did not count: rather than studying the social condition of humanity in total, social theory was exclusively about the social condition of men. In response to these criticisms, attempts have been made to include women in the purview of social theory. However, these often simply involve going on in the same old way but tagging a chapter on women on at the end. I am aware that this chapter might seem to be an instance of this sort of begrudging strategy. I hope it is not. While I feel the theoretical positions of feminisms are sufficiently important to warrant a separate treatment in the form of a chapter, I have also attempted to introduce feminist issues throughout the book, such as Celia Davies' critique of occupational roles in Chapter 2 and Anne Witz's analysis of professional strategies in Chapter 4.

Even more at odds with traditional social theory is postmodernism, which explicitly rejects the possibility of progress, upon which most social theorising has to date been based. Instead of seeking to gain a true and adequate picture of social reality, along with a blueprint for the way in which reality could be improved, postmodernists argue that there is no one way of looking at social reality and that the assumption that there is leads to social tyranny as believers in a particular perspective seek to force their interpretation upon the rest of us. As an alternative to the striving for an adequate understanding of the world, postmodernists celebrate differences of opinion.

9 Feminisms, caring and women's knowledge

Introduction

One of the main difficulties I encountered in writing this chapter was what to include and what not to include. As there are many forms of feminism, inclusion of them all was not possible. However, at the same time, I wished to give some recognition to the diversities of feminism. As a result, I opted for a compromise. In order to demonstrate diversity, the chapter starts with a brief discussion of three traditionally strong strands of feminism – liberal feminism, Marxist feminism and radical feminism. I then concentrate in depth on two branches of feminism that have particular salience to nursing. The first is cultural feminism, which I explore through the work of Carol Gilligan (1982), using as a nursing example Winifred Pinch's (1994) study of care for women with HIV/AIDS. The second approach is that of standpoint feminism, interrogated largely through the work of Hilary Rose (1986) and linked to nursing through Elizabeth Hagell's 'Nursing knowledge: women's knowledge' (1989).

The development of feminist approaches

One way in which to examine feminisms is to view their development as an increasing disenchantment with mainstream (or, in feminist terminology, 'malestream') social theory. From a belief that women's autonomy could be incorporated within the logic of Enlightenment thought, feminists have become increasingly sceptical about the capacity of even critical sociological approaches to give due account to women's understandings and experiences. This has led to the construction of radically alternative approaches to social theorising. The bulk of this chapter will deal with these approaches. However, in order to see how feminist thought arrived at such a position, we will start with a brief review of the historical trajectory of feminisms, starting with liberal feminism.

Liberal feminism

As its name suggests, liberal feminism is grounded in liberal political thought, which itself adheres to the central tenets of Enlightenment thought (see Chapter 7). Basically, classical liberalism is founded upon the assumption that the uniqueness of human beings rests upon rationality: our ability to use reason to understand the world is what distinguishes us from other species. Based on this premise, liberal political thought asserts the importance of individuals' rights to exercise their reason without hindrance. They therefore advocate a political system that promotes individual autonomy. Moreover, all people, by virtue of their human rationality, have a right to this autonomy; as a result, liberalism underlines the importance of equal rights.

Liberal feminism has a long pedigree, stretching back over two centuries to Mary Wollstonecraft's *A Vindication of the Rights of Women*, (1970 [1792]). Wollstonecraft attacked the assumption that women were naturally less reasonable and more emotional beings than men. She argued that differences between the sexes in the areas of reason and emotion were the result of social circumstances. She likened the middle class women of her day to caged birds, who spent their days confined to the home, preening and pluming themselves. Their social confinement within the male-dominated family meant that women were denied health, liberty and virtue. Because they were prevented from going outdoors (in order to keep fashionably pale), women were unable to exercise and therefore lacked healthy bodies. Because the male head of the family made all important decisions in the family, women lacked liberty. Because the use of education to develop rationality was largely confined to boys, women were discouraged from developing their powers of reason and therefore lacked virtue (reason being the ultimate virtue).

For Wollstonecraft, the way out of the bird cage was through equality of education for women and men. A real education would allow women to sharpen their minds and develop their reason. Women could then use that rationality to act autonomously. This would, of course, involve an alteration in the nature of family relations, women being allowed to make decisions for themselves, becoming equal partners rather than a 'toy of man, his rattle' (1970: 34).

Basically, Wollstonecraft's argument was that if women had equal rights and opportunities, they would be able to develop as equals to men. The problem here is that she 'presents us with an ideal of female education that gives pride of place to traits traditionally associated with males at the expense of others traditionally associated with females' (Roland Martin 1985: 76). One of the consequences of this celebration of rationalism is that it fails to examine critically traditional male modes of thought. As we shall see, these become a central target for later feminists.

I would not like to give the impression that liberal feminism is simply a historical footnote. It remains alive and well to this day and has indeed been at the forefront of demands for both educational and legal reforms that have given women a more equal place in society. Probably the best known contemporary liberal feminist, whose book *The Feminine Mystique* (1963) did much to launch the second wave of feminism in the USA, is Betty Friedan. Friedan argues that women are ensnared by the feminine mystique, which is the idea that they can find satisfaction in their traditional roles of housewife and mother. Condemned to the dissatisfying drudgery of household chores, smothering their children with obsessive-compulsive love and denied meaningful goals in life, women lead empty lives. For Friedan, escape from this emptiness lies in women gaining education and using that education in full-time public work. Rather than being the whole of her life, marriage and motherhood would then only be one aspect, allowing her to fulfil herself in the goal-directed, creative activity of paid work. This may sound all well and good, but as any nurse who is also a mother will attest, the effort and sacrifice required to keep all these roles going simultaneously is not inconsiderable. Moreover, it would appear that, for Friedan, the meaningful goals that women should aspire to are defined according to male definitions of success.

Marxist feminism

While liberal feminists argue that the way forward is to reform the system so that women can enjoy the same opportunities as men,

Marxist feminists argue that because it is the system – capitalism – that causes women's oppression, reforms will not solve the problem. Instead, what is required is an overthrowing of capitalism.

As with liberal feminism, Marxist feminism is grounded in a distinct theoretical tradition (see Chapter 3). However, its basic assumptions about the nature of humanity differ radically from those of liberalism, which, you will remember, asserts that the uniqueness of human beings rests upon their rationality. In contrast, Marxists believe that our 'species being' involves our capacity to mould the world to our own ends through labour. Through their collective activities, men and women create society, which in turn shapes them. Within capitalism, the type of society with which we are faced is both exploitative and alienating. Moreover, Marxist feminists argue that it is even more exploitative and alienating for women than for men.

To illustrate the positions that Marxist feminists take, I will briefly review three arguments about how capitalism oppresses women. The first is that of Marx's close colleague, Friedrich Engels, in a book entitled *The Origin of the Family, Private Property, and the State* (1985 [1884]). Engels saw the oppression of women as being the result of the institution of private property, as it had been developed by capitalism. Men, as the group that leave the private sphere of the family to engage in labour and commerce, are the ones who accumulate private property (why it should be men who go out, Engels is not too clear about). As a result, the economic order of the family reflects the economic order of society, the man being the propertied bourgeois, the woman the propertyless proletarian. This oppressive relationship is exacerbated by the desire of men with property to ensure that it is passed on to their own children. Because the identity of a child's father has (until recently) been an uncertain matter, the institution of compulsory monogamy for women was introduced. The monogamous family, for Engels, did not come about because of love or friendship but because of economic imperatives. Engels was not behind the bush in clarifying the demeaning effects that the family had on women:

> This marriage of convenience often enough turns into the crassest prostitution – sometimes on both sides, but much more generally on the part of the wife, who differs from the ordinary courtesan only in that she does

not hire out her body, like a wageworker, on piecework, but sells it into
slavery once and for all.

(Engels 1985: 79)

For Engels, the first stages of emancipation for women would
involve their wholesale return to the public workforce and the
socialisation of housework and child care (in other words, turning
them into tasks that are done by collectives of people rather than
by individuals on their own, as is done within families).

The second example of Marxist feminist thinking that I wish to
address is that of Eli Zaretsky (1976), who argues that while patriarchy (male dominance in the family or in wider social spheres) pre-
dated capitalism, capitalism made matters considerably worse for
women. Prior to the rise of capitalism, most work was carried out
within the family or, at its widest, within the local community.
Clothes-making, furniture production, child care, building, farming
and cooking were all carried out by family members. As a result,
women were intimately involved in the labour process.

With the advent of capitalism, all this changed. Production
moved out of the household and into the factories. Because of pre-
existing patriarchal structures, it was the men who now went out
to work and women who stayed behind to mind the household.
This had a momentous effect upon gender relations:

Capitalism is the first society in history to socialize production on a large
scale. With the rise of industry, capitalism 'split' material production
between its socialized forms (the sphere of commodity production) and
the private labour performed predominantly by women within the home.
In this form, male supremacy, which long antedated capitalism, became
an institutional part of the capitalist system of production.

(Zaretsky 1976: 29).

Given that male supremacy is institutionalised within capitalism, the only way to overcome it and gain an equal position for
women in society would be through the overthrow of capitalism.
In Zaretsky's words, 'The family cannot be transformed except as
part of the general transformation and destruction of the capitalist
economy' (1974: 93).

The two examples that I have used so far have tended to
emphasise the oppression that emanates from capitalism rather than

from men (perhaps this is because they were both written by men!). Other Marxist feminists have been less 'economistic' (economism being the approach that attempts to explain all social phenomena in terms of economic relations). Instead, their task has been to cure Marxism of what they see as its gender blindness through an examination of how gender relations both relate to and differ from economic relations. Thus, our third example, Michèle Barrett, defines the object of Marxist feminism in the following terms:

> In the most general terms, it must be to identify the operation of gender relations as and where they may be distinct from, or connected with, the processes of production and reproduction understood by historical materialism... In this context a Marxist feminist approach will involve an emphasis on the relations between capitalism and the oppression of women. It will require an awareness of the specific oppression of women in capitalist relations of production, but this must be seen in the light of gender divisions which preceded the transition to capitalism and which, as far as we can tell, a socialist revolution would not of itself abolish.
>
> (Barrett 1980: 9)

Using these three examples, I have attempted to give an idea of the spectrum of Marxist feminist thought, ranging from a fairly crude 'capitalism causes women's oppression' type of argument (Engels), through a more subtle 'capitalism may not have caused women's oppression, but it perpetuates it' thesis (Zaretsky), to the assertion that capitalist oppression and the oppression of women are two different, although connected, processes (Barrett). For some feminists, Barrett's qualification, which still accepts the significance of class to women's oppression, does not go far enough. These feminists are often grouped under the label 'radical feminists'.

Radical feminism

For radical feminists, it is gender relations rather than class relations that generate fundamental inequalities in the social world. For them, women's oppression is the oldest, the most widespread, the most obdurate and the most extreme form of oppression that exists between humans (Jagger and Rothenberg 1984). Therefore, attempts to understand and eradicate oppression should use as their basis gender divisions rather than economic ones.

The difference between Marxist feminism and radical feminism is most graphically demonstrated in Shulamith Firestone's *The Dialectic of Sex* (1979), in which she attempts to turn Marx on his head. In her examination of the patriarchal oppression of women, Firestone takes the *form* of historical materialism but changes the *content*. Instead of economic class divisions being the driving force of her dialectic, as it was in Marx's, Firestone points to what she calls 'sex class divisions'. Thus, she reformulates historical materialism as:

> that view of the course of history which seeks the ultimate cause and the great moving power of all historical events in the dialectic of sex: the division of society into two distinct biological classes for procreative reproduction, and the struggles of these classes with one another.
>
> (Firestone 1979: 12)

Here, Firestone is asserting the importance of reproduction, in contrast to Marx's emphasis on production. In turn, because human reproduction is fundamentally a biological matter while production is fundamentally an economic matter, Firestone argues that the roots of women's oppression are biological rather than economic. The struggle thus becomes one between the class that controls the means of reproduction (men) and those who lack control (women). Just as in Marx's class struggle, liberation requires revolutionary action by those who currently lack control:

> So that just as to assure elimination of economic classes requires the revolt of the underclass (the proletariat) and... their seizure of the means of *production*, so to assure the elimination of sexual classes requires the revolt of the underclass (women) and the seizure of control of *reproduction*.
>
> (Firestone 1979: 19)

The most obvious objection to this point of view might be that while economic arrangements can be changed, at least in principle, as a result of human actions such as socialist revolution, biological arrangements are not amenable to such actions. Firestone does not accept this and points to the ever-increasing capacity of technology to change and control biological functions (think for example of contraceptives or in vitro fertilisation).

Firestone argues that reproductive technologies could be harnessed to eliminate the biological basis of women's oppression by freeing women of their exclusive role as childbearers:

> The reproduction of the species by one sex for the benefit of both would be replaced by (at least the option of) artificial reproduction: children would be born to both sexes equally, or independently of either, however one chooses to look at it; the dependence of the child on the mother (and vice versa) would give way to a greatly shortened dependence on a small group of others in general... The division of labour would be ended by the elimination of labour altogether (through cybernetics). The tyranny of the biological family would be broken.
>
> (Firestone 1979: 19)

An ambitious project you might say. Perhaps too ambitious. It is not simply a matter of whether or not technology will get to the point at which it is able completely to take over both human reproduction and human labour. It is also a matter of the role that technology plays in our society. You will remember from Chapter 7 that one of the primary concerns of critical theorists was the increasing engulfment of our lives by a 'technocratic consciousness', which threatens to drown human freedom and autonomy altogether. For critical theorists, Firestone's technological utopia would be the very epitome of hell.

Challenging difference

While the feminist approaches that I have discussed thus far contain considerable differences, they have at least one characteristic in common: they all play by the established rules of the game of social theory. By this, I mean that, in calling for the full inclusion of women in the social world, they frame their demands in terms that are compatible with the discourses that have already been established by male social theorists. Thus, liberal feminists argue that the values of individual freedom and equal rights should be extended to fully include women; Marxist feminists use the insights of political economy as a point of reference for their analysis of women's oppression; and even Firestone uses the intellectual tools developed by Karl Marx to posit her theory of the dialectic of sex.

Whether they see changes in the law or in economic or technological arrangements, all of these theorists seek an end to the differences that foster women's inequality: they wish to see the development of a common humanity, in which no-one is disadvantaged on account of their sex. In short, they all fall within the tradition of the Enlightenment and its aspiration for a rational and humane ordering of society.

Cultural feminism

Not all feminists are convinced that the aim of ending differences between women and men is a viable or even desirable goal. Instead of aspiring to human sameness, cultural feminists accept that there are differences between the sexes and celebrate the unique culture of womanhood. As Judith Evans notes, cultural feminism is characterised:

> by its insistence that women's characteristics and values are for the good, indeed are superior and ethically prior to men's, and should be upheld. They and certain of women's roles (for various writers, motherhood would be a case in point) have been derogated, devalued, by men. It is part, anyway, of feminism's task to revalue them, to reclaim woman's heritage, or woman's pride.
>
> (Evans 1995: 76)

One of the areas of difference that has been interrogated by cultural feminists is that of moral reasoning – the different ways in which women and men approach moral problems. This issue was brought to prominence by the psychologist Carol Gilligan in her formulation of the feminine ethic of care.

The ethic of care

The ethic of caring has been identified by feminist nursing commentators as central to the work of nursing. Thus, for example, Jean Watson identifies 'the basic core of nursing as comprising the philosophy and science of caring' (1979: xv), while Madeleine Leininger states that 'caring is the central and unifying domain for the body of knowledge and practices in nursing' (1981: 1). What I wish to do in this section is to examine how the issue of caring, so salient to the occupation of nursing, can be placed in a more general discourse about the nature of women's moral reasoning.

Carol Gilligan's seminal work *In a Different Voice* (1982) was written in response to the orthodox views in developmental psychology concerning the supposed lack of moral development displayed by girls. The implications of this view, which stretched back to Freud, were that women were unable to think objectively or to get beyond particular concerns in order to apply general principles to moral problems. Gilligan, while accepting that there were differences, did not accept that they indicated deficiencies in women's moral reasoning. Instead, she argued that the attributes of women's moral reasoning, which do not assert general principles to the cost of particular concerns or seek absolute, 'objective' standards that may be of little relevance to the instances in which they are invoked, are strengths rather than weaknesses (Evans 1997).

The evidence Gilligan uses for her argument comes from a number of different sources. I will discuss just one source here, namely her reinterpretation of experimental interviews with two children, a boy and a girl, originally devised by the psychologist Lawrence Kohlberg to test his theory of the stages of moral development.

The two 11-year-olds, Jake and Amy, were presented with a dilemma. They are asked to place themselves in the position of 'Heinz'. Heinz's wife is dying, but there is a drug that could save her life. However, Heinz is unable to afford the drug, and the pharmacist refuses to lower its price. The dilemma is: 'Should Heinz steal the drug?'

Jake is quite clear that Heinz should indeed steal the drug. He methodically runs through the rationale behind his decision, arguing that human life is more important than money, that the pharmacist could replace the losses caused by the theft but that Heinz could never replace his wife. Asked about the fact that, in stealing, Heinz is breaking the law, Jake confidently asserts that laws cannot cover all instances, and that, if caught, he would expect the judge to be lenient with Heinz. When asked how he worked his way though the moral dilemma presented to him, Jake replies that it is 'sort of like a math problem with humans'. In contrast, Amy's reply to the question of whether Heinz should steal the drug appears far less sure:

Well, I don't think so. I think there might be other ways besides stealing it, like if he could borrow the money or make a loan or something, but he really shouldn't steal the drug – but his wife shouldn't die either.

(quoted by Gilligan 1982: 26)

When asked why she thinks that Heinz should not steal the drug, Amy does not talk about property rights or the law against stealing but of the effect that the theft would have upon Heinz's relationship with his wife:

If he stole the drug, he might save his wife then, but if he did, he might have to go to jail, and then his wife might get sicker again, and he couldn't get more of the drug, and it might not be good. So, they should really just talk it out and find some other way to make the money.

(quoted by Gilligan 1982: 28)

Gilligan argues that instead of seeing the dilemma as a 'math problem with humans', Amy sees it as a problem with relationships. Stealing would simply threaten the relationship between Heinz and his wife and, as a result, threaten her life. Moreover, the aspect of the dilemma that really puzzles her is the attitude of the pharmacist, arguing that if Heinz were to communicate with the pharmacist to point out the consequences of his refusal to lower the price of the drug, the pharmacist would realise that he should give the drug to the wife and arrange for Heinz to pay for it later. In this solution, we can once again see the emphasis Amy places on relationships.

In assessing the responses of the two children, the researchers involved came to the conclusion that Amy was a full stage below Jake in her moral development. They came to this conclusion on the grounds that she was unable to think systematically about moral concepts and was reluctant to challenge authority or question received moral truths. Gilligan puts an altogether different interpretation on Amy's responses, which, because it encapsulates her thesis about the strength of women's moral reasoning and its connection with the ethic of care, I will quote at length.

Her world is a world of relationships and psychological truths where an awareness of the connection between people gives rise to a recognition of responsibility for one another, a perception of the need for response. Seen in this light, her understanding of morality as arising from recognition of relationship, her belief in communication as the mode of conflict resolution, and her conviction that the solution to the dilemma will follow from its compelling representation seem far from naïve or cognitively immature. Instead, Amy's judgements contain the insights central to an ethic of care, just as Jake's judgements reflect the logic of the justice approach. Her incipient awareness of the 'method of truth', the central tenet of nonviolent conflict resolution, and her belief in the restorative activity of care, lead her to see the actors in the dilemma arrayed not as opponents in a contest of rights but as members of a network of relationships on whose constitution they all depend.

(Gilligan 1982: 30)

Gilligan thus contrasts the male moral point of view as an ethics of justice with the female moral point of view, which she describes as the ethics of care. Thus, for men, the moral imperative is to respect the rights of others; for women, the moral imperative is to care – to identify and alleviate the troubles that affect themselves and others. Fully developed, the ethics of care involves neither selfishness or self-sacrifice but a realisation of the connectedness of human beings.

Before moving on to a nursing example of the ethic of care, I would like to make a qualifying point about cultural feminism. One of the dangers of taking such an approach is that it can lead to an absolute equation that woman = caring and man = instrumental. This approach is termed 'essentialism', in that it assumes that these different approaches are part of the essence of what it is to be female or male. The objection to this formula is that men can be caring and women can use masculine ethics, such as formal justice. Reflecting this problem, Celia Davies has argued that we should talk instead of 'cultural codes of masculinity and femininity [which] will map, but not neatly, on to real people' (1995: 30). This notion of cultural codes allows us to be more subtle and flexible in our analysis.

Nursing example: women and AIDS

A good example of how nurses might practically utilise the ethic of care is to be found in a paper by Winifred Pinch entitled 'Vertical transmission in HIV infection/AIDS: a feminist perspective' (1994). Pinch argues that Gilligan's model of the way in which women process moral dilemmas can inform both nursing assessment and nursing actions.

For women who have HIV-positive children through vertical transmission (from infected mother to child via placenta or breast milk), the moral dilemmas to be faced are not inconsiderable. In many cases, whether or not she has a partner, the woman will have sole responsibility for the care of the child. There is a need to deal with both her own condition and that of the child. The woman will have to consider her own terminal illness, which may mean that she will die before the child. She may have to make separate arrangements for the child if she becomes too ill to engage in child care herself. This then leads to complex questions relating to extended family support or the option of foster care. Given these huge dilemmas that many women with HIV/AIDS face, Pinch identifies three main approaches to nursing actions that can facilitate and empower women through the promotion of connectedness and care.

The first of these nursing actions is the obtaining of HIV-infected women's 'psychological profiles' (to use Pinch's own, rather scientific, terminology) in order to assess the degree of stress, anxiety, depression and isolation from which they are suffering. Pinch notes that women, as a systematically oppressed group, are more likely anyway to experience stress and anxiety. However, given the specifics of HIV infection, which is often associated with maladaptive social contacts, such as the sharing of needles or unprotected sexual activity, women with HIV/AIDS may seek to isolate themselves, using strategies such as secrecy or denial to help them cope with their illness. This lack of connectedness will only increase their stress. As a result, one of the purposes of exploring women's feelings is to enable the nurse to help her patients to overcome isolation strategies, thus enhancing their social connectedness.

As Pinch notes, social connectedness does not simply have the effect of enhancing psychological well-being. Thus, for example, a study of women with breast cancer clearly indicated that women involved in supportive group therapy not only had less anxiety and depression, but also lived longer and suffered less pain (Spiegel et al. 1989). Reflecting this insight, the second nursing action identified by Pinch is that of group therapy. This can have two related benefits. On the one hand, it allows women to find their voice and, through telling their story, to integrate the events they have experienced into their life history. On the other hand, the 'resonance one may hear with other women's stories can be affirming, encouraging, empowering' (Pinch 1994: 41). Once again, we can clearly see the twin themes of caring and connectedness.

The final nursing approach identified by Pinch is the promotion of self-esteem:

> The self-esteem of a woman should also be a nursing concern. High self-esteem is necessary for assuming responsibility (read power) for reproductive decisions. Power as dominance is not necessarily a goal for women. However, women need to be empowered to make choices and select decisions that sustain the critical relationships in their lives. The challenge is to support caring and nurturing behaviour, while enhancing self-esteem and self-confidence so that desirable activities are fully understood and freely chosen.
>
> (1994: 42)

The aim, therefore, of the nursing care of women with HIV/AIDS is first of all to come to an understanding of 'where women are' currently and then to develop strategies of interventions that will help them to cope with future situations. This becomes especially important in cases where the woman has an HIV-positive child because this entails acute moral dilemmas around the areas of connection and responsibility.

Feminist epistemology

The issue of caring and its relation to women's work is not restricted to moral reasoning: it also has ramifications for epistemology (how and in what way we know about things). Here, a feminist approach, known as 'standpoint feminism', has attempted to uncover how knowledge, particularly scientific knowledge, is inherently gendered. However, before examining what standpoint feminism involves, we need, in order to get a theoretical background, another excursion back to Marxism, this time to the ideas of the Hungarian Marxist, Georg Lukás (1885–1971).

Lukás and praxis

Lukás (pronounced loo-cash) came from an odd pedigree for a Marxist thinker. Prior to World War I, his writings were strongly anti-positivist, being influenced by writers such as Weber. It was not until the war that he turned to Marxism, and even then he maintained a strongly anti-positivist stance, which was considerably at odds with the orthodox scientific Marxism of his day. In his major work, *History and Class Consciousness* (1971 [1923]), Lukás' target was the mechanical view of the social world that saw historical change as the result of iron laws and that relegated human consciousness to an effect of those laws. This view entailed the assumption that the meaning of history was to be understood through scientific explorations of the objective structures of capitalism (here we can see echoes of Durkheim in Chapter 1 and structuralism discussed in the introduction to Part III). Lukás rejected this, arguing that in order to understand historical developments, it is necessary to turn to the consciousness of the working class.

His basic argument was that the inferior *social* position of the working class actually provided its members with a superior *epistemological* position. Because of their oppression, they were able to come to know the nature of capitalism and its evils far better than were the bourgeoisie, who benefited from current arrangements. The proletarian has a coherent understanding of the social world, because she is, in Lukás' terms, both subject and object. On the one hand, the proletarian has an awareness of her exploited position in society, which, by extension, gives her a knowledge of the overall arrangements pertaining. In short, she is a knowing subject. On the other hand, capitalist economic relations reduce the proletarian to the status of a commodity, a thing to be exploited, denying her fundamental humanity. Thus, we have proletarian as object. When the proletarian becomes aware of her situation, subject and object unite, society is grasped in its 'totality', and actions are taken to challenge the object status that capitalism inscribes upon workers.

The central point Lukás is making is that human consciousness is far more than a mere effect of external conditions. History moves in the way it does as a result of human actions, and those actions come about on the basis of the understandings of actors. Conversely, in acting upon the world and changing it, actors gain a fuller understanding, which will in turn condition future actions. Class consciousness and revolutionary practices (knowledge and action) are therefore two sides of the one coin, a relationship that is summed up in the term *praxis*.

To summarise, while proletarian Marxists share the same world with the bourgeoisie, they understand that world in radically different ways as a function of their differing social positions. Bourgeois thought takes current reality as a natural given; because the bourgeoisie enjoys great benefits within the *status quo*, it does not see the possibilities of alternatives, and views change with fear and trepidation. In contrast, proletarian thought, because it is in the interests of proletarians to abolish capitalism, has a better understanding of the underlying dynamics of system. For Lukás, then, proletarian thought stands on a higher plane than bourgeois thought.

Standpoint feminism

Just as Shulamith Firestone used Marxist analysis of the relations of production between economic classes and substituted relations of reproduction between sex classes, so standpoint feminists take the Marxist analysis of praxis and class consciousness and apply it to gender consciousness. Thus, the following statement by Hilary Rose could almost be taken from *History and Class Consciousness*:

> Real knowledge is history from below. It is not merely a question of achieving a balanced view of the world, but of transformative knowledge imbued with an understanding of the dynamic of history – the history of humanity and the history of nature.
>
> (Rose 1986: 162)

However, for Rose, the working class does not have the uniquely privileged position that Lukás ascribes to it. Rose also wishes to include the standpoint of women's knowledge as providing a more adequate form of understanding than masculine forms of knowledge.

Accepting the notion of praxis, Rose argues that human knowledge comes from practice, from working on and changing the world. What makes humans unique compared with other species is that their efforts to alter the world to their own ends is guided by consciousness rather than instinct. Rose concludes from these observations that 'science is organized knowledge of the world derived from practice upon it' (1986: 162). Because science is based upon labour, it is shaped by the purposes of that labour. The practice from which science is derived is a practice that seeks to control and master nature and humanity. Here we can discern clear echoes of the critical theory argument discussed in Chapter 7, which stated that science, rather then being concerned with understanding *per se*, is used as an instrument to control and manipulate nature. The difference here is that standpoint feminists regard this controlling science as being peculiarly masculine.

The feminist historian Londa Schiebinger (1989), in tracing the relationship between gender and science, argues that while women were not initially seen as incompatible with scientific activity, they had by the start of the nineteenth century been successfully squeezed out through a process of both institutional and ideological exclusion. Women then had an uphill struggle to fight their way back in, a struggle that continues to this day. However, this is not simply a matter of individual women being prevented from following scientific careers. Because they were excluded during a crucial and prolonged period in the development of the scientific community, they had little part to play in the construction of the scientific project. As a result, the forms of scientific understanding that pertain today are to a large degree the product of male practice (Evans 1997). From the perspective of standpoint feminists, those forms of understanding are far from edifying:

> Masculinist knowledge takes the form of a peculiar emphasis on the domains of cognitive and objective rationality, on reductive explanation, and on dichotomous partitioning of the social and the natural worlds. It is this masculinist knowledge which has produced today's deadly culture of science and technology and which seeks to relegate women and women's knowledge to the realm of nature.
>
> (Rose 1986: 162)

In other words, the scientist is seen as divorced from the world, using his rationality to uncover the objective truth about it. That objective truth tends to reduce the complexities of the world to simple relations of cause and effect. The natural world and human culture are seen as two separate and distinct aspects of reality, and while men are placed in the area of culture (and are therefore seen as being able to shape their destiny, culture being the result of human activities), women are regarded as being controlled by their nature or biology and therefore lacking in human autonomy.

We might think here, as an example, of a middle-aged women going to her male GP, complaining of low self-esteem and depression, which he interprets as being caused by hormone imbalances and therefore prescribes hormone replacement therapy. In doing so, he fails to ask her what *she* feels is the cause of her depression, a course that could well uncover explanations for her low self-esteem in the social or personal circumstances she is experiencing.

What of women's labour and women's knowledge? The first thing to note is that women's labour is exploited and undervalued. Here we come back round to the activities involved in caring for others. As Rose points out, women's labour is a combination of long hours of menial labour, which is boring and repetitive (think of housework), and complex emotional work with children, husbands and elderly people. All of these practices are seen as unskilled and are therefore not rewarded in terms of either social status or financial remuneration. The emphasis on the superiority of objective scientific knowledge means that the experiential knowledge, intuitive abilities and emotional complexities involved in caring are simply discounted. Worse, they are exploited for the benefit of men – the time spent by women engaging in housework and child care frees up time that men would otherwise need to dedicate to maintaining themselves and their progeny. Thus, ironically, men can only engage in the activities that they value because they exploit those activities performed by women, while at the same time discounting the importance of women's activities (Bologh 1990).

Take, for example (an entirely hypothetical example, you understand), a male academic writing a book on social theory and nursing practice. Discovering that he has made a total mess of his time management, he realises that he is going to have to work 15 hours a day, 7 days a week for a month, if he is going to stand any chance of meeting his publisher's deadline. So, instead of vacuuming, cleaning toilets or minding the kids, he spends all his time sitting in front of his personal computer bashing out great profundities. However, all those activities of housework and child care still have to be performed, book deadlines or no, so his partner has to take up the slack. But who gets the credit for the book? Certainly not the person who has spent her precious time doing household tasks and caring in order that the academic might gain the time to write it.

Here we can see how, in the exploitation of their labour by men, women are reduced to the status of objects, to use Lukás' terminology. But women are also knowing subjects. Caring may often be a form of exploited labour, but that does not mean that, in certain circumstances, it is neither pleasurable nor fulfilling. While women's caring exists predominantly in an alienated form (alienation is discussed in Chapter 3), there are glimpses of non-alienated caring, which is freely given without coercion and which provides the signposts for how future social relationships might be constructed. Moreover, women's activities provide them with a framework of knowledge that is qualitatively different and, as standpoint feminists would have it, truer and more complete than masculinist knowledge:

> feminist epistemology derives from women's lived experience, centred on the domains of inter-connectedness and affectual rationality... Such an epistemology transcends dichotomies, insists on the scientific validity of the subjective and the need to unite cognitive and affective domains; it emphasizes holism, harmony and complexity, rather than reductionism, domination and linearity.
>
> (Rose 1986: 162, 179)

In short, women's standpoint within society enables them to have a knowledge of the totality of social and natural relations that men, by virtue of their privileged position, are unable to grasp. Instead of regarding the world as something out there that is to be controlled and manipulated, feminist epistemology understands that the knower is connected to that world (both natural and social) through a myriad of binding threads. Moreover, it does not reduce knowledge to cold, purposive rationality but accepts that feelings and values, including the feelings and values of others, are also part of rationality.

While starting out from a Marxist framework, standpoint feminists have moved the issue of knowledge into realms far beyond those envisaged by traditional Marxists. They have challenged the assumptions of social theory in general by exposing its overweening emphasis on analyses and actions based on cognitive rationality. Put another way, social theory, being largely a male practice, has promoted male ways of knowing. The aim of standpoint feminism is to introduce female ways of knowing into social discourse. However, for some feminists, the standpoint position does not go far enough, in that by positing a 'right' way of approaching knowledge, it censors out other possibilities, other voices. These feminisms adhere to postmodernism, which will be the subject of the next chapter (although it will not interrogate the specific lens of feminist postmodernism).

Nursing example: nursing knowledge, women's knowledge

One of the most eloquent pleas for women's knowledge to be used as the foundation for nursing knowledge can be found in Elizabeth Hagell's 'Nursing knowledge: women's knowledge' (1989). In her own words, her article:

> attempts, by using sociological and feminist theory, to support the idea that nursing has a distinct knowledge base which is not grounded in empirico-analytic science and its methodology but which stems from the lived experiences of nurses as women and nurses involved in caring relationships with their clients.
>
> (Hagell 1989: 226)

Hagell traces the rise of medical science, linking it to the rise of male domination in capitalist society. She argues that nursing developed in the way in which it did in response to the requirements of male medics for cheap and obedient labour to perform menial health care tasks, in order to maximise their profits. In terms of knowledge, it was male medicine that made all the running, establishing positivist science as the only valid form of health care knowledge. Thus, we return to Evans' (1997) point that because women were excluded from the scientific community for so long, the forms of scientific understanding that pertain today are to a large degree the product of male practice. While nursing has been attempting to break into the charmed circle of established health care professions, it has, until recently, been forced to do this by playing the rules of the game already established by male medicine in medicine's interests. In other words, nursing has imitated medicine's use of science in the construction of its knowledge base.

However, there has in recent years been an increasing questioning of the assumptions involved in the scientific approach, and attempts have been made by theorists such as Leininger to develop a different approach to nursing knowledge that puts more emphasis on caring as its central component.

You will remember Rose's point that knowledge is not context free but derives from practice. Hagell argues that the problem currently facing nursing is that while nursing practice is largely based on the ethic of care, nursing theory remains, to a large degree, in the thrall of scientific approaches. 'This incongruency results in an increasing distance between belief and action and leads to confusion, despair and frustration' (Hagell 1989: 230). The way to establish a congruency between nursing theory and nursing practice is to establish the space whereby practice can inform theory. In other words, there is a need to incorporate knowledge based upon the ethic of care into nursing theory. Using the work of Watson (1985), Hagell identifies a more appropriate focus for nursing knowledge:

> nursing knowledge may be defined as knowledge of people (or people in groups) and health–illness experiences that are mediated by human care transactions. It allows a close and systematic observation of one's own experience and seeks to disclose and elucidate the lived world of human health–illness experience and the phenomena of human-to-human caring.
>
> (Hagell 1989: 231)

Hagell does not advocate the complete abandonment of scientific approaches. However, she does argue both that it should no longer be the dominant intellectual framework and that it should be opened to constant critical examination.

Hagell provides a number of practical suggestions as to how nursing can go about establishing and promoting its own forms of knowledge. Key to these are changes in nursing education. She advocates that nursing curricula should include critical evaluations of nursing theory, utilising alternative modes of thought such as feminism, Marxism and critical theory (given the nature of this book, I can only say bravo). She also argues that critical courses on the history of nursing, which expose the social and political influences upon the occupation's development, should be introduced. Central to changes in education would be the introduction of feminism:

> This would rekindle the lost emphasis on caring. It would also make nursing education a political education in the sense that it would illuminate power relations that exist in society and within the health care system.
>
> (Hagell 1989: 231)

Feminism would also need to be incorporated into nursing research, to be used as a theoretical basis for research investigations. Conversely, Hagell argues that, until recently, the women's movement has paid little attention to nursing. She advocates that links between nurses and women active in the women's movement should be widened and strengthened.

The importance of Hagell's argument lies in her linkage of women's knowledge with nursing knowledge. To put it in Lukás' terms, she is arguing, first, that nurses have been constructed as objects by their medical colleagues. However, their role as carers, while involving a socially subservient position, enables nurses to be knowing subjects, and provides them with the capacity to see health and health care in its totality rather than confining it to the narrow realm of technical interventions in response to physiopathologies.

The significance of accepting difference

The significances of standpoint and cultural feminisms are twofold. First, their rejection of aspirations to sameness with men and their celebration of women's differences means that they present us with radically different views of morality and knowledge, questioning taken-for-granted notions of justice and rationality. In doing so, they challenge the foundations of much of social theory, which has largely been characterised by male concerns.

The second, related, significance is that, if accepted, these feminisms hold out the promise of providing nursing with the theoretical bases for a radical re-evaluation of knowledge and practice. They offer us a caring practice that can hold its head up as providing a more holistic approach to the problems of human health than that of masculine science, and a nursing knowledge that is firmly grounded in that practice.

Recommended further reading

In terms of feminisms in general, a very useful introduction is provided by Rosemary Tong in her *Feminist Thought* (1989). If you wish to sample the writings of feminist theorists, both Maggie Humm (1992) and Miriam Schneir (1995) provide well-chosen readers. To see how feminist issues connect with nursing, you could do no better than refer to Celia Davies' *Gender and the Professional Predicament in Nursing* (1995). Finally, in line with Hagell's recommendations, feminist concerns have increasingly come to animate nursing research during the 1990s, although this has been a far from unproblematic process. An example of the tensions that exist between feminist principles and the strictures of conforming to scientific procedural rules of research, along with a discussion of how the medical establishment can undermine nursing research, is to be found in Jennifer Mackenzie and Christine Webb's 'Gynopia in nursing practice' (1995). A fine critique of the construction of women as governed by their biology, and the positing of an alternative feminist construction of female sexuality, can be found in Cheryl Few's (1997) paper on sexual health work with young women.

10 Postmodernism and Foucault

Introduction

Once again, this chapter is funnelled. It starts with a general discussion of some aspects of postmodernist theory and how it distinguishes itself from modernism. This is largely done through an examination of the ideas of Jean-François Lyotard. The chapter then moves on to the work of Michel Foucault, his theories concerning the relationship between knowledge and power, and how those theories might be used to illuminate health care relations. To show how Foucault's theory of knowledge can be applied to nursing issues, I review Julianne Cheek and Trudy Rudge's (1994) examination of nursing discourse as found in case notes. In relation to his notions of power and surveillance, I turn to Michael Bloor and James McIntosh's (1990) study of the surveillance activities of health visitors.

However, before starting, I should warn you that pinning down just what postmodernism means is an extremely difficult task, if only because one of the central tenets of postmodernism involves the argument that we can never pin down what anything really means. However, a clue to its approach is found in the word itself, which implies that it is about something that comes after (post) modernism. Given that it defines itself in relation to modernism, we should start by trying to untangle what that term means.

Modernism

First of all, where does the term 'modern' come from? In literal terms, it is derived from the Latin for 'of today'. However, that is not much help, in that anyone living at any time in history could describe themselves as 'of today' at that time, and indeed, the term 'modern' has been used at a number of junctures in history. However, its current use is more specific than this and derives from the great Enlightenment thinkers of the seventeenth and eighteenth centuries (see Chapter 7) who made the distinction between the *anciens*, who wished to hold on to the theological certainties of the medieval world, and themselves, the *modernes*, who wished to move forward to freedom based on rationality. With the French Revolution, and its clarion cry of *liberté, egalité et fraternité*, modernity emerged from the world of ideas and into the social domain. The key concepts here are rationality and progress. Rather than relying on the providence of God, Enlightenment modernists argued that human beings could use their own rationality to ensure progress in the world towards the realisation of freedom, equality and community. As we have seen so often during this book, this concept of rationality was closely connected with science and the technological capacities based upon science; the promise of modernity was not only to make us free, but to make us comfortable as well.

However, the trajectory of modern progress has been far from an easy ride; for all the pros of modernity, we can also identify profound cons. Thus, in the realm of science, set against the development of synthetic insulin is the development of the atomic bomb; in the realm of economics, set against the development of the welfare state is mass starvation in Africa; in the realm of politics, set against the French revolutionary cry for freedom is the swish of Monsieur Guillotine's blade.

This same ambivalence can be found in the realm of social theory. If we take the three founding fathers of Part I, each of them, in their different ways, had their worries about the nature of modernity. Durkheim, for all his belief in social solidarity, accepted that such solidarity was threatened by the nature of modernity. You will remember from Chapter 2 his identification of 'organic solidarity' as the form of social organisation in the modern world. With organic solidarity, collectively held values and beliefs become less important than they were in the medieval world. In their place arises the morality of individualism, which asserts the importance of the individual over and above that of the social group. Durkheim believed that the emphasis on the individual entailed by organic solidarity posed a profound threat to the cohesion of society but argued that this problem could be overcome by the development of a new form of moral regulation (Durkheim 1964).

As we saw in Chapter 3, Marx was also a great believer in the possibility of progress, seeing the development of modern capitalism as a way-station to the freedom and comfort of communism. However, Marx was also acutely aware of the social and intellectual maelstrom that capitalism entailed:

> Constant revolutionizing of production, uninterrupted disturbance of all social conditions, everlasting uncertainty and agitation distinguish the bourgeois epoch from all earlier ones. All fixed, fast-frozen relationships, with their train of ancient and venerable prejudices and opinions are swept away, all new-formed ones become antiquated before they can ossify. All that is solid melts into air, all that is holy is profaned.
>
> (Marx and Engels 1967: 83)

Yet Marx believed that out of this chaos a solid and universal system of justice could be built. He argued that the proletariat had the capacity to build a classless society, which would entail a system of justice that would not be based upon the vested interests of one section of society, as had been the case in all previous class societies (Daly 1996).

Weber was by far the most pessimistic of the founding three. You will remember the rather apocalyptic quotation in Chapter 7 from his *The Protestant Ethic and the Spirit of Capitalism* (1930), in which he identifies the iron cage of modernity, populated by specialists without spirit and sensualists without heart. For Weber, the 'progress' of modernity was of very dubious value. It is hardly surprising then that of these three theorists, he is the one most favoured by postmodernist thinkers.

Leaving Weber aside, we can see how both Durkheim and Marx identified problems with modernity as they found it, but posited directions by which society could overcome those problems. As such, they remain within the spirit of the Enlightenment, in that they applied a rational critique of the conditions facing them and, on the basis of that critique, offered a path of further progress.

Postmodernism

The problem for postmodernists is that these paths of progress did not lead where their architects expected them to. In terms of

Durkheim, time has seen societies becoming even more fragmented and individualised than they were in his day. A new form of moral regulation has simply not materialised. As far as Marx is concerned, just as the French revolution led to the guillotine, so the Russian revolution led to the mass murders of Stalin.

It is not just that postmodernists reject the notion of progress on the grounds that it is an unrealisable dream (although they certainly do take this position). It is also that they argue that these dreams of progress will always end in tears. Trying to squeeze humanity, in all its diversity, into the confines of an overarching model, or 'metanarrative' as Jean-François Lyotard (1984) terms it, inevitably leads to the subjugation of those who do not fit in with our ideas of the way forward. For postmodernists, the rise of Stalin was not a tragic warping of the ideals of Marxism but rather part of the logic of the Marxist metanarrative, which led to violent attempts to subjugate the autonomy of individuals in the name of proletarian progress.

Postmodernists argue that Enlightenment attempts to overcome the divisions between social groups through the identification of common, universal bonds should be abandoned. They argue that society is characterised by difference rather than totality: there is no social whole out there waiting to be realised at the end of the yellow brick road of progress. Attempts to force people down that road simply lead to terror:

> The nineteenth and twentieth centuries have given us as much terror as we can take. We have paid a high enough price for the nostalgia of the whole and the one, for the reconciliation of the concept and the sensible... The answer is: Let us wage war on totality;... let us activate the differences.
>
> (Lyotard 1993: 46)

More succinctly, Lyotard says elsewhere, 'Simplifying to the extreme, I define *postmodern* as incredulity towards metanarratives' (1984: xxiv). This means that almost all the knowledge claims that we have discussed thus far become suspect. It is not just a matter of the debunking of science. (We have seen how others, such as Husserl – Chapter 5 – with his argument that positivist science failed to recognise the active nature of human consciousness, and the critical theorists – Chapter 7 – with their critique of the use of science to dominate nature and humanity, have tried to do the same thing.) Equally for postmodernists, Husserl's claims that the phenomenological method can gain us access to the authentic self, and critical theory's attempts to return to a more value-oriented rationality, are regarded as dangerous fictions. Thus, Lyotard attacks Habermas' aspiration for communicative action (Chapter 7) on the following grounds:

> Is legitimacy to be found in consensus obtained through discussion, as Jürgen Habermas thinks? Such consensus does violence to the heterogeneity of language games. And invention is always born of dissension. Postmodern knowledge... refines our sensitivity to differences and reinforces our ability to tolerate the incommensurable. Its principle is not the expert's homology, but the inventor's paralogy.
>
> (1984: xxv)

First, let me define some of these rather cumbersome terms. Heterogeneity means diversity and incongruousness, incommensurable refers to the absence of a common standard of measurement or judgement, and homology means taking the same position, while paralogy means taking a position contrary to reason. Thus, what Lyotard is arguing is that the way in which different people interpret the world is often incongruous with the interpretations of others (heterogeneity). By attempting to get them to interpret the world in the same way (homology), we warp those interpretations. Rather than seeking to achieve such a goal, postmodernism happily accepts that there are many ways of looking at the world and that there are no standards by which to judge which of these ways is better than the others (tolerating the incommensurable). Indeed, if we did all agree in our interpretations, our lives would lack all dynamism and inventiveness, because it is only through challenging accepted reason that anything novel is ever produced (hence postmodernism's embrace of paralogy).

In traditional philosophical terms, postmodernist theory is 'relativist', relativism being the belief that different ways of knowing (science, Buddhism, magic, scientology, animism, whatever) are simply that – different. They can be adjudged neither better nor worse than each other because there are no rules or procedures for deciding what is 'truth' and what is not. As a consequence, we have no access to 'reality', and 'reality', whatever it is, does not impinge upon our interpretations.

Foucault and knowledge

Having given a very brief outline of one or two aspects of postmodernism through the lens of Jean-François Lyotard, I now wish to move on to issues more pertinent to health through the examination of the work of Michel Foucault (1926–84), who, while sitting somewhat uncomfortably within the postmodernist genre, is the theorist of that style who has had most impact upon nursing discourse. For the sake of clarity, I am going to divide up my treatment of Foucault into two parts, the first concerning his treatment of knowledge and the second concerning his treatment of power. This is an artificial division, in that the assumption that knowledge and power are inseparable was central to Foucault's work. However, as we run through the discussion, I hope that this relationship will become clear.

Foucault's aim in his treatment of knowledge was to challenge modernist, Enlightenment assumptions about its nature. The first modernist assumption that we will address is that knowledge can be understood in its own terms, that it can be judged true or false through the observation of the reality it purports to explain, and the use of rationality to clarify and explain our observations.

Let me take a practical example of our (modernist) notion of the way in which knowledge works. If I say to you that Mr Jones has a urinary tract infection, you can go and examine his urine to see whether it is foul smelling and cloudy. Moreover, to be certain, you can send it to the laboratory to test whether it contains bacteria. On the basis of your own observations and rational interpretation of those observations and, even more persuasively, your acceptance of the scientific expertise of the medical laboratory scientific officer who analyses the specimen, you can be fairly certain of whether or not my interpretation of Mr Jones' urine reflects its real condition. This all sounds very straightforward – these sorts of procedure for testing whether we have an adequate interpretation of what is really going on are part of our second nature. However, this very term 'second nature' indicates the issue concerning Foucault: we assume that the way in which we go about knowing things is the natural way, without considering the many assumptions that lie behind our knowledge or pondering to think that people in other cultures and times have interpreted cloudy urine in many different ways. What is it about our assumptions that makes us go straight for the bacteriological answer?

These are the types of question that Foucault asks, and it is on the basis of his answers that he rejects the notion that knowledge can be treated in its own terms. Rather than approaching statements of fact by attempting to judge their truth, Foucault asks 'how is it that one particular statement appeared rather than another?' (Foucault 1974: 27). What conditions make certain kinds of knowledge possible? After all, if you lived in a society or a time when people did not think in terms of bacterial infection, my statement that Mr Jones had a urinary tract infection would then make no sense to you at all. Foucault argues that, while we are rarely aware of it, we all operate with a set of common assumptions about the nature of reality, which provide the basis for our conscious knowledge. He terms these sets of common assumptions 'discourses', which he contrasts with our usual conception of knowledge in the following terms:

> discourse is not a slender surface of contact, or confrontation, between a reality and a language... [I]n analysing discourses themselves, one sees the loosening of the embrace, apparently so tight, of words and things, and the emergence of a group of rules proper to discursive practice. These rules define not the dumb existence of a reality... but the ordering of objects. [The task] consists of not – of no longer – treating discourses as groups of signs... but as practices that systematically form the objects of which they speak.
>
> (Foucault 1974: 48–9)

What Foucault is saying here is that he wishes to go beyond the question of whether knowledge or language provides an adequate representation of reality. Knowledge does not simply consist of the application of linguistic or mathematical signs that describe reality, as the correspondence theory of truth that we came across in Chapter 6 would have it. Instead, knowledge actively orders reality in certain ways, doing so on the basis of the assumptions that make up the 'discursive formation' within which the knower is located. There is no one true way of knowing about things. Instead, there are innumerable ways of ordering the chaotic events that occur so that they make sense to us. Our belief that the rational and scientific procedures we use to order and interpret events are obviously the correct approach is simply an illusion.

The second modernist assumption that Foucault questions is that of the progress of knowledge. Modernists assume that, over time, our knowledge of reality has become more accurate. Thus, for example, the advent of science gave us a better description of what is going on in the world than did medieval religion. Foucault uses his identification of discursive formations, upon which knowledge depends, to undermine the modernist image of rational scientific progress, which sees knowledge marching ever onward towards a 'truer' and more detailed grasp of reality. He regards such notions of the incremental progress of science as invalid justifications for the tyranny of what he terms 'totalising discourses' (an alternative term to Lyotard's metanarratives). Instead, he sees the history of ideas as one of discontinuity, which results from radical shifts in the underlying discursive formations rather than improvements in knowledge (Foucault 1970).

This argument rests upon his disconnection of knowledge and reality, mentioned above. If knowledge and reality are not related, we have no grounds for judging whether one set of beliefs about the world is more valid than another:

> 'Effective' history differs from traditional history in being without constants. Nothing in man – not even his body – is sufficiently stable to serve as the basis for self-recognition or for understanding other men.
>
> (Foucault 1991: 87)

This historical relativity, with its assumption that one interpretation of the body cannot claim superiority over another, has the effect of undermining the knowledge claims about the body of contemporary health care sciences. Thus, Foucault compares two descriptions of illnesses, one from the eighteenth century and one from the nineteenth. While the nineteenth-century account has a familiar ring to it, the earlier description seems quite bizarre to the twentieth-century reader:

> membranous tissues like pieces of damp parchment... peel away with some slight discomfort, and these were passed daily with urine; the right ureter also peeled away and came out whole in the same way... the oesophagus, the arterial trachea, and the tongue also peeled in due course; and the patient had rejected different pieces either by vomiting or by expectoration.
>
> (Foucault 1976: ix)

Foucault's point in making this comparison goes further than observing that there are differences in perception over time. It entails the assumption that there is no way of deciding which perception is better. To underline this, Foucault poses the question: 'How can we be sure that an eighteenth-century doctor did not see what he saw?' (1976: x). If we follow Foucault, we have to accept that modern conceptions of the body and ways of caring for it are no better than previous conceptions; they are simply different.

As we have seen, when combined, Foucault's critiques of the modernist assumptions that knowledge can be understood in its own terms and that knowledge has progressed through history add up to a refutation of a third assumption that some descriptions of reality are truer than others, irrespective of their social or cultural context. Indeed, if we go with Foucault, reality comes in danger of fading our of the picture altogether, in that he regards our notions of reality as simply the creation of discourses. This line of argument can clearly be seen in Foucault's discussion of the work of the nineteenth-century postmodernist *avant la lettre*, Friedrich Nietzsche (1969 [1887]), in which Foucault contends that attempts to uncover the essence of reality are doomed to failure:

> This search [for origins] is directed to 'that which was already there', the image of a primordial truth fully adequate in its nature, and it necessitates the removal of every mask to ultimately disclose an original identity. However, if the genealogist refuses to extend his faith in metaphysics, if he listens to history, he finds that there is 'something altogether different' behind things: not a timeless essential secret, but the secret that they have no essence or that their essence was fabricated in a piecemeal fashion from alien forms.
>
> (Foucault 1991: 78)

These alien forms are the result of discourses, which are in turn the expression of power relations. The influence of power relations upon our construction of the world is one of Foucault's central themes. He argues that: 'power produces reality; it produces domains of objects and rituals of truth. The individual and the knowledge that may be gained of him belong to this production' (Foucault 1977: 194). As a result, if we wish to understand the history of knowledge, we need to understand how that knowledge has been produced by power. Foucault terms this way of going about history 'genealogy'.

The ability of power to produce reality results from the intimate relationship between power and knowledge: 'There is no power relation without a correlative constitution of a field of knowledge, nor any knowledge that does not presuppose and constitute at the same time power relations' (Foucault 1977: 27). This sounds rather forbiddingly philosophical. Basically, what it means is that knowledge is never used simply for the sake of understanding the world. Rather, it is always used and constructed with a purpose in mind. That purpose may either be to control nature or to influence the behaviour of others. Hopefully, this idea of the close relation between knowledge and power will become clearer after we have worked through an example of the connections between power, knowledge and discourse.

Nursing example: nursing as textually mediated discourse

The relationship between power and knowledge in nursing discourse has been interrogated in a paper by Julianne Cheek and Trudy Rudge entitled 'Inquiry into nursing as textually mediated discourse' (1994). What Cheek and Rudge hope to show in this paper is that nursing knowledge does not simply mirror the reality of health care encounters. Rather, it actively constructs that reality using assumptions that are embedded within the discursive framework of medicine. Furthermore, this construction of reality reflects and reinforces the power relations that exist between health care workers and their clients.

Cheek and Rudge examine hospital case notes through a postmodern variant of discourse analysis. This approach goes beyond discourse analysis' usual concentration on the technical aspects of textual language, to examine how those texts are part of the construction of nursing reality. Cheek and Rudge base their analysis on Van Dijk's Foucauldian (the 'd' instead of a 't' is not a mistake but reflects French grammar) approach to discourse, which sees it as 'a system of statements which cohere around common meanings and values... [that] are a product of powers and practices, rather than an individual's sets of ideas' (Van Dijk 1990: 231). They also note that at any one point in time, various discursive frameworks will coexist. Some will complement each other, others oppose each other; some will be dominant, others submerged within that dominance.

The study involves discourse analysis of the case notes of two randomly chosen patients: Mr H, a 64-year-old man who has suffered a debilitating stroke, and Mrs W, who has fractured her femur, both having been admitted into a rehabilitation unit. The first thing that Cheek and Rudge note is that the discursive frameworks of science and medicine powerfully shaped the construction of the case notes:

> Both Mrs W and Mr H were represented by chemical notations, blood count results, and other forms of symbols. The language used was objective and the tone depersonalized. The documentation of other health professionals follows the medical form of examination or assessment, plans, prescribed actions, and timelines for evaluation. The use of highly specialized and technical language by the medical staff effectively denies access to the uninitiated, including the individual who is technically constructed by the notes.
>
> (Cheek and Rudge 1994: 62)

Thus, the scientific discourse of medicine enjoys a powerful position on two counts. First of all, because other health professionals, including nurses, adopt the voice of medicine, its discourse has the power to shape the knowledge of those professions with which it works. Second, because the language used is inaccessible to those about whom it is written, patients have no opportunity to affect this discourse and therefore the construction of their reality as patients. Thus, the power of medicine is reinforced by its exclusive access to knowledge.

Cheek and Rudge examine the rituals of admission, which both reinforce and at the same time mask to the patients the power relations that exist between the patients and the professionals. These rituals serve to establish the 'reality' of the patients' condition and thus legitimate their entry into care. In the process, patients are reduced to their illnesses. Thus, Mrs W is represented by the admitting physician as: 'D: # R) NOF' (Cheek and Rudge 1994: 63), and Mr H as 'D: R) CVA' (1994: 63). While using slightly more accessible notation, the admitting nurse reflects the medical objectification of patients in her contribution to the notes, describing Mrs W as 'a fall who had fractured her femur' (1994: 63).

The personal experience and knowledge of the patients is notably absent from the case notes, which were almost exclusively dominated by the rational scientific voice of medicine. Even when the voice of the patient is recorded, the validity of the claims made by the patient are not accepted until they can be verified in terms of scientific knowledge. Thus, for example, the notes record that Mrs W 'claims she can't see out of her right eye'. As Cheek and Rudge comment:

> Until it can be verified objectively and in the scientific/medical voice, it is a debatable point whether or not Mrs W can see. Her personal knowing, her reality, is effectively discounted and instead takes on that which is being textually mediated for her. In fact, the personal experience and knowledge of the individual concerned is systematically expunged from the case notes.
>
> (1994: 63)

The case notes also indicated that nurses were prepared to be extremely authoritarian in ensuring that their version of reality, rather than the patient's, was adopted as valid. Consider the following entry, which reports on an attempt by Mrs W to get out of bed to use the commode, which was not successful, resulting in her being incontinent on the floor: 'Nurse passing her room heard scraping furniture and investigated the noises, *rescued* the patient and *reprimanded* her... the client was *reminded* that ...' (Cheek and Rudge 1994: 64). Similarly, following an incident in which Mr H fell, the nursing report stated: 'Patient *instructed* to ring bell if he wants anything and not to get out of bed unaided. Seems *compliant* with order' (1994: 64). These reports do not simply reflect the reality of the dangers that confronted these patients and the nursing response to those dangers. What is crucially absent from these accounts is any sense of Mrs W or Mr H's personal experiences and interpretations of their situation. The nurses' reality is imposed upon them, the tone of the case notes implying that clients must accept the reality that has been constructed for them by health care workers and that they will be reprimanded if they fail to do so.

So far, we have reflected on how patients' interpretations of reality are obliterated from the construction of reality in clinical case notes. However, Cheek and Rudge also address how nurses' constructions of reality, which do not fit in with the authoritarian, scientific discourse of medicine, are undermined. Thus, they recount an entry by a speech therapist reporting that nursing staff have informed her that Mr H's wife is having considerable emotional difficulties. However, information about these difficulties are not documented by the nurses themselves, who leave it up to other health care professionals to decide whether this information is significant enough to merit reporting. Instead, nurses tend to report on the more trivial aspects of their caring role, such as the time until which Mr H watched television. This example demonstrates how, in their construction of reality in the case notes, nurses fail to write in their own unique contribution to health care interactions. As Cheek and Rudge note, this self-denial is consonant with Pearson and Baker's assertions about nursing documentation:

> nursing judgements are not valued by either the nurse[s] who make them or their peers. If the indications of this study are valid, this must also apply to the tasks that they carry out... most of what nurses write is data which are valued by medical, paramedical and administrative staff. They [nurses] are not capturing their own effectiveness in their documentation.
>
> (1992: 47)

We can see from Cheek and Rudge's paper how health care knowledge is neither a straightforward reflection of reality nor innocent of power. The knowledgeable statements produced by the nurses in the case notes reflect the assumptions of medical discourse, and that discourse is in turn produced by and reproduces the unequal power relations that pertain between health care professionals and their clients.

Foucault and power

While, in the previous section, we have examined how power produces knowledge, we have not really considered what Foucault means when he talks of power. It is to this issue that I now wish to turn. Foucault's notion of power is considerably different from traditional interpretations. I will briefly examine four aspects of his approach, as formulated in the first volume of his *History of Sexuality* (1979), that demonstrate the novelty of his conception of power.

First, Foucault argues that power cannot be explained in terms of social structures or institutions. It is not a matter of one group, be they the bourgeoisie, men, the government or whoever, having power over the rest. Rather, he sees power as being generated at the point of interaction between individuals:

> I do not have in mind a general system of domination exerted by one group over another, a system whose effects, through successive derivations, pervade the entire social body. The analysis, made in terms of power, must not assume that the sovereignty of the state, the form of the law, or the over-all unity of a domination are given at the outset; rather, these are only the terminal forms that power takes. It seems to me that power must be understood in the first instance as the multiplicity of force relations immanent in the sphere in which they operate and which constitute their own organization.
>
> (1979: 92)

Thus, while Foucault does not deny the existence of social and institutional power, he sees them as being derived from the interactions of individuals: 'Power comes from below; that is, there is no binary and all-encompassing opposition between rulers and ruled at the root of power relations' (1979: 94).

Second, rather than seeing power as something that is possessed by certain persons or groups, and not by others, Foucault characterises it as part of the process of interaction:

> Power is not something that is acquired, seized, or shared, something that one holds on to or allows slip away; power is exercised at innumerable points, in the interplay of nonegalitarian and mobile relations.
>
> (1979: 94)

What he is saying here is that it is not a matter of some people having power (whether or not they are using it) and others not. Power only comes about during interactions between people, when those interactions, as they invariably do, display relations of inequality. This is going even further than Giddens' assertion (Chapter 8) that social structures only have a virtual existence until they are 'instantiated' by action. Here, even virtual existence beyond instances of interaction is denied structured power relations.

Third, Foucault challenges the idea that power is only exercised in certain circumstances, or that it is possible to enter into relations that are not tainted by power. Instead, he argues that the exercise of power is extremely widespread. For Foucault, power is omnipresent 'because it is produced from one moment to the next, at every point, or rather in every relation from one point to another. Power is everywhere... because it comes from everywhere' (1979: 93).

This is not to say that power relations involve the unproblematic domination of one person by another. For Foucault, the exercise of power always provokes resistance. Thus, the fourth aspect of his definition of power is that power and resistance are two sides of the same coin: 'Where there is power, there is resistance, and... this resistance is never in a position of exteriority in relation to power' (1979: 95).

Panoptic surveillance

Having examined the nature of power, we now need to address how relations of power operate in contemporary society. Foucault (1977) argues that the modern period saw the birth of new forms of power that were far more invasive than anything seen before. In his own terms, power relations now take the form of 'panoptic surveillance'. Panopticism literally means 'seeing everything'. Foucault took the term 'panopticon' from the nineteenth-century English philosopher and social reformer Jeremy Bentham, who used it to describe a model prison that he had designed. The novelty of this prison was that, instead of throwing prisoners into a dungeon where they would be out of sight and out of mind, prison cells were arranged in such a fashion that their occupants could all be seen from a central guard post. The prisoners in the panopticon could never tell whether or not they were being watched, so they had to behave at all times as if they were. As a result, Bentham argued, they would reform their behaviour.

Foucault argues that this sort of surveillance is endemic throughout society. When we go to school, we are monitored to see whether we are polite and diligent; when we go to work, we are monitored to see whether we keep to time and are sufficiently productive; and, as we shall see, when we seek health care, we are expected to behave in certain, well-defined ways. Indeed, matters are worse than this because, just like the prisoners in Bentham's panopticon, we realise that we may be being monitored at any time, so we behave at all times as if we are. In other words, we survey ourselves, acting as our own moral wardens, a process that Foucault describes as 'subjectification' (Rabinow 1991).

What is the aim of all this surveillance? The answer to this question is well summed up by Merquior, who clearly illustrates Foucault's affinity to Weber's analysis of modern life, and the iron cage to which it condemns us:

> The web of discipline aims at generalizing the *homo docilus* [docile man] required by 'rational', 'efficient', 'technical' society: an obedient, hard-working, conscience-ridden, useful creature, pliable to all modern tactics of production and warfare. And ultimately the main way to achieve docility is the moral pressure of continuous comparison between good and bad citizens, young or adult: discipline thrives on '*normalizing judgement*'. Bourgeois society bred an obsession with the norm, from the 'écoles normales' to the keeping up of standards in industrial production and the concern with general norms of health in the modern hospital.
>
> (Merquior 1991: 94)

These 'normalising judgements' are made by experts in the human sciences, such as teachers, judges, social workers, physicians, psychiatrists and nurses, who use their professional knowledge to define what is classed as normal, who fits into this definition of normality and what is to be done with those who do not fit in.

To summarise Foucault's argument thus far, power relations in contemporary society largely consist of the surveillance activities of experts who monitor our behaviour or personal attributes, decide whether these fit into their definition of normality and act upon us if they do not. Perhaps at this point we need a practical example to illustrate what this 'obsession with the norm' entails.

It is a true story, with due apologies to Ewan, who will probably never forgive me after he learns to read this. In August 1992, I was blessed with child, a son who weighed in at a not inconsiderable 9 lb. In the dubious manner of the traditional Irish male, I was extremely smug about having fathered such a fine strapping lad, but I had not reckoned on the power of the expert. Ewan was hardly out of the womb before he was placed under intense surveillance, the aim of which was to ascertain whether or not he fitted the experts' definition of what passed as normal for a neonate. Using her knowledge, in the form of a statistical table, and her (rather basic) technology in the form of a tape measure, the midwife quickly came to the conclusion that, lying in the fifth decile for height, Ewan was not normal. He was too tall.

This decision put in train a whole series of consultations and procedures, involving midwives, general practitioners, health visitors and eventually a consultant paediatrician. Cognitive tests were performed and blood samples taken. In short, the medical panopticon was marshalled in all its glory in order to ascertain the cause of this breach of normality. Fortunately, the story has a happy ending. I was not present at the first consultation with the paediatrician, who, in rather vague terms hinted that abnormal height could be a sign of genetic pathology. I was, however, present at the second consultation, when we were informed that blood tests had not come up with any evidence of genetic problems. I noticed that the paediatrician kept looking at me in an odd fashion. Eventually she said, 'I'm beginning to think that things are probably fine. I had been concerned about both his height and his dysmorphia. However, now you are all together, I think it's only a matter of family resemblance. However, it would probably be a good idea that we continue to monitor him.' At this point, the power of surveillance provoked our resistance – the suggestion of further monitoring was politely but firmly refused. As an aside, it is too painful to explain the meaning of dysmorphia; all that I will say is that the paediatrician was very lucky that I did not work it out myself until after I left her office.

The clinical gaze

In *The Birth of the Clinic* (1976), Foucault focuses specifically on the manner in which medical surveillance is carried out. He argues that the reality of the patient is constructed by what he terms the 'clinical gaze' of physicians. Under the clinical gaze, the patient becomes a body to be manipulated, reduced to the pathologies that she displays. Moreover, conceptualised through the medium of anatomical atlases, the body is seen as nothing more than a biological machine. The signs and symptoms of that machine are compared with what the expert 'knows' about normal anatomy and physiology, and, using this knowledge, the physician decides the possibilities of restoring the pathologised body to normality and acts accordingly.

Foucault's critique of the way in which the clinical gaze reduces patients to objects is not novel. Think back, for example to Chapter 7 and Scambler's (1987) Habermasian portrayal of how the medical experts fail to take account of the lifeworld experiences of their clients. One of the results of critiques of this nature has been a refocusing of health care practitioners, not least nurses, on personal and individual care. However, it will be remembered that Foucault sees power in all relationships, and relationships involving individualised care are no exception.

Pastoral power

Late in his career, Foucault developed the notion of 'pastoral power', which, in contrast to the clinical gaze, is a form of surveillance that directs itself towards people as individual subjects rather than as objects, and which 'implies a knowledge of the consciousness and an ability to direct it' (Foucault 1982: 214). Carl May has argued that the development of individualised care in nursing is a prime example of the exercise of pastoral power, noting that:

> nurses are now required to extend their 'gaze' beyond the concrete condition of the body, and to intrude into the patient's private, *subjective* sphere... Here 'knowledge' about the patient follows from the notion that her clinical disassembly [her reduction to machine status under the clinical gaze] has had the effect of mystifying her 'real' or 'authentic' character, and that this can be reinstated through 'talking', 'listening', or 'counselling' in which this whole person or individual may be brought into view.
>
> (1992: 591)

The problem here is that, while the clinical gaze reduced people to their bodies, at least its surveillance was limited to those bodies. In contrast, by adding our psyche and our social circumstances to the gaze of health care workers, pastoral power widens the trawl of surveillance to the most intimate parts of our lives. Thus, another Foucauldian commentator, David Armstrong, characterises the development of holistic, individualised care in nursing as follows:

the nurse is now instructed to communicate with the patient as a subjective being: the patient must confess and the nurse must listen. The nursing process, for example, offers a pervasive analysis and constant awareness of the patient's (and nurse's) personal worlds... From a simple concern with the care of the patient's bodily functions, nursing has started to become a surveillance apparatus which both monitors and evinces [reveals] the patient's personal identity: in doing so it helps fabricate and sustain that very identity.

(1983: 459)

Nursing example: the surveillance of health visitors

In a study entitled 'Surveillance and concealment' (1990), Michael Bloor and James McIntosh use a Foucauldian perspective to uncover both the surveillance activities of health visitors and the strategies of resistance to that surveillance adopted by working class Glasgow mothers. Building on the idea of pastoral power, they develop the concept of the 'therapeutic gaze'. This surveillance technique, which parallels the clinical gaze, constitutes people as psychosocial beings and involves the observation, interpretation and redefinition of their behaviour.

Bloor and McIntosh start by identifying the role of health visiting, which, they argue, involves a preventative service that both monitors the physical and emotional well-being of babies and infants, and encourages healthy lifestyles and parenting practices. They note that surveillance is central to the role, most obviously in the health visitor's obligation to monitor evidence of abuse or neglect. However, they argue that the surveillance functions of health visitors are more pervasive than this. Specifically, they are sceptical of health visitors' claims that, in their health education role, they are non-directive and non-judgmental. Health education is not neutral but contains a set of values that may or may not be shared by health visitors' clients. Those values entail assumptions about what is 'good' and what is 'bad' parenting, what is a 'healthy' and an 'unhealthy' lifestyle. The aim of health visiting is to persuade parents to conform to the standards that are valued by health visitors. In short, health visiting involves the promotion or maintenance of those behaviours regarded as appropriate. One of the consequences of this is that health visitors need to know whether the behaviour of parents accords with their prescriptions. This information can only be attained through surveillance. Using Foucault's (1979) connection of knowledge and power, Bloor and McIntosh state that:

> Professional knowledge – like all knowledge – is never disinterested: immanent in the discourse of health visiting are relations of power; power and knowledge are always intermingled... Non-directive professional advice is thus a chimera, or perhaps a strategy of influence in itself.
>
> (1990: 163)

However, health visitors are not all-powerful wardens of child care. It will be remembered that Foucault (1979) argued that the exercise of power always provokes resistance. Bloor and McIntosh identify a number of strategies of resistance adopted by mothers in the face of health visiting surveillance. They term the first strategy 'individual ideological dissent'. This involves mothers challenging the legitimacy of health visiting discourse, in the belief that child care is a skill that is learned through experience rather than theoretical learning. Thus, one of the mothers interviewed by Bloor and McIntosh stated:

> Half the people who try tae tell ye aboot weans (children) have no' got weans o' their own. Ah mean, they're just readin' off books an' that. Ah prefer tae go tae people that's got experience. Ah mean, they just laugh at them up there (clinic). A health visitor wi' nae kids trying tae tell a woman that's got five what tae dae?
>
> (quoted by Bloor and McIntosh 1990: 172)

The second form of resistance involves hidden non-compliance with health visitors' advice. In other words, if they were offered advice with which they disagreed, mothers would accept it politely and then promptly go on to ignore it:

> ye just agree wi' her (health visitor) and do yer own things 'cause she's no here every day to check.
>
> (1990: 174)

Thus, for example, much against the health visitors' advice that solid food should not be introduced to babies before 4 months, 40 per cent of the babies in Bloor and McIntosh's sample were weaned by 6 weeks.

The third strategy was escape or avoidance, which involved mothers either stopping clinic visits or avoiding contact with the health visitor in the home. The fourth strategy involved conceal-ment and deception. This had advantages over avoidance in that it neutralised the power of the health visitor without the risk of confrontation. Here, it was not simply that the mothers listened and then ignored advice but rather that they actively constructed inaccurate accounts of their behaviour:

> Ah tell them what they want tae know. Ah mean, she widnae be very pleased if she kenned we had him on solids when he was two weeks old. But ye don't tell her that. She'd do her nut. Ye say, 'Oh no, he's just having his milk'.
>
> (1990: 176)

Bloor and McIntosh's study has the merit of alerting us to the fact that relationships between health care practitioners and clients inevitably take the form of power relations. In turn, those power relations are closely bound up with knowledge claims. On the one hand, health visitors use their professional knowledge base to define what 'normal' parenting is and use tactics of surveillance to ascertain whether those standards of normality are being adhered to by their clients. On the other hand, mothers have their own, less formal knowledge base about appropriate ways to bring up children and adopt various strategies of resis-tance to minimise the inequalities of power that exist in their rela-tionships with health visitors.

Conclusion

To bring the discussion back round to postmodernism, it can be seen how Foucauldian approaches to knowledge deny that there is any one way of understanding the world that is intrinsically better than other ways. The reason why some perspectives, notably science, have gained such prominence is not because they are epistemologically privileged but because they are successfully imposed through the exercise of power. Knowledge is not a matter of getting to know the world better; rather, it is part of the 'will to power', to use Friedrich Nietzsche's (1968 [1901]) term. This will to power can be seen in all social relationships. This in turn means that progress is an illusion; the development of democratic political forms, for example, has not led to a reduction in the exercise of power but rather to its further diffusion – while the King used to tell us what to do, it is now the health visitor.

This may all seem very novel, and indeed postmodernists revel in their novelty and their capacity to debunk taken-for-granted verities. However, at this point I want to take you back to the start of this book. You may remember that Chapter 2 commenced with a discussion of the seventeenth-century philosopher, Thomas Hobbes. There, I quoted Hobbes' portrayal of the condition in which humans would find themselves without social order: 'they are in that condition which is called Warre; and such a warre, as is of every man, against every man' (1968: 185). Compare this to a quotation from Michel Foucault:

> This is just a hypothesis, but I would say it's all against all. There aren't immediately given subjects of the struggle, one the proletariat, the other the bourgeoisie. Who fights against whom? We all fight against each other.
>
> (Foucault 1980: 208)

The postmodernist message is thus that modernist attempts to solve the problem of social order have failed and will indeed never succeed. Progress towards a rationally organised society is merely a dangerous illusion that has been used to justify the barbarities of those who believe they know the way forward.

Social theory is founded on the assumption that it is possible rationally to explain social reality and, in doing so, point to weaknesses in the forms that society takes. Thus, it at least implicitly points the way to progress. Given these underlying assumptions, the acceptance of postmodernism entails the rejection of the whole *raison d'être* of that which passed before it, making much of this book, along with many others, redundant.

However, not all social theorists have accepted Foucault's diagnosis. Many, including myself (Porter 1996a, 1996b), have argued that while power is important, the total collapse of knowledge into power is just as unconvincing as the naïve modernist belief that knowledge can be totally innocent of power. To take such a position leaves open the possibility of rational critique and social progress. The debate goes on, but it is here that we must leave it.

Recommended further reading

For an in-depth, although sometimes rather difficult, application of postmodernist ideas to the field of health, see Nicholas Fox's *Postmodernism, Sociology and Health* (1993). In relation to nursing, a favourable assessment of the use of postmodernism can be found in Lister's 'The art of nursing in a "postmodern" context' (1997), while a critique can be found in Kermode and Brown's 'The postmodernist hoax and its effects on nursing' (1996).

For accessible treatments of Foucault, you could turn either to Barry Smart's *Michel Foucault* (1988) or the considerably less favourable *Foucault* by J.G. Merquior (1991). As I mentioned above, the merits and demerits of Foucault in relation to nursing have also caused some debate. The main lines of argument are encapsulated in a paper that I wrote with the Australian Foucauldian scholar, Julianne Cheek, in which she presents the case for Foucault, while I present the case against (Cheek and Porter 1997).

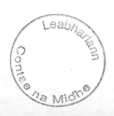

AFTERWORD

We have now come to the end of our tale. By way of an afterword, let us take stock of our efforts. I think the first thing to note is that this book is a tale. By this I do not mean that I simply made it all up. What I do mean is that the book provides just one of many possible stories that could have been written about social theory. Now, I happen to think that the approach that I have taken was a reasonably coherent way of ordering my subject matter. It started with an examination of the foundations of social theory, moved on to a strand of theory that is becoming increasingly dominant in research of nursing practice, then looked at attempts to synthesise social theory and finally considered attempts to construct entirely new theoretical projects. However, as I have said, the book could have been completely different in form and just as coherent. For example, rather than concentrating on different schools, I could have looked at social theory through the substantive areas that it addresses, with chapters on such topics as power, progress, gender, class and bureaucracy. In many ways, it is simply a matter of taste, and this was my taste.

Decisions had to be made all the way down the line on what should go in and what should be left out of the book, and I am afraid that a lot had to be left out. To take just two examples of recent developments in social theory that are of considerable pertinence to nursing practice, I have not included examination of the sociology of risk, which has come to the forefront of social theory since the publication of Ulrich Beck's *Risk Society* (1992), nor have I addressed the burgeoning sociology of the body that owes much to the foundational work of Bryan Turner (1996).

Nor is it just a matter of leaving out whole areas of theory. Even within those areas which I have addressed, many important schools and contributors have been totally ignored. Thus, for example, in our look at phenomenology, we did not discuss hermeneutics at all, avoiding mention of the important works of Hans-Georg Gadamer (1975) and Paul Ricoeur (1966). Similarly, the increasingly influential postmodern feminists such as Luce Irigaray (1985) fell between the stools of cultural and standpoint feminisms on one side and male postmodernist theorists on the other. Even my identification of the three 'founding fathers' is open to dispute. For example, Ian Craib (1997), in his recent text on classical social theory, adds George Simmel to the triumvirate.

Of course, if all these theorists (and the many more that do not even get a mention in this qualification) had been included, we would be talking about a book of several volumes. I had to make a call about whom to leave in and whom to neglect. I made it on the basis of two main criteria. The first was the pertinence of the theoretical approach to nursing concerns. Thus, for example, while action theories were favoured with an entire part to themselves, structuralism was not so blessed. Second, on the grounds that a textbook should provide its readers with a grounding in the basic aspects of a discipline, I favoured those theories that were reasonably established within the sociological corpus, steering clear of theoretical approaches that are just in the process of development, which is why I have omitted risk theory and the sociology of the body.

The final thing I want to do is to take a tentative look into the future: what might social theory look like in the medium term? We saw in Chapter 10 that the whole project had come under intense pressure from postmodernism's rejection of progress and celebration of difference. However, as I mentioned at the end of that chapter, the battle between modernism and postmodernism in social theory is far from over – we need only look to the increasing vibrancy of critical realism. Nor do I feel that it will ever be decisively concluded. Indeed, had we wished, we could have constructed the entire history of social theory (not to mention the whole of philosophy) around the continual swing between belief in the possibility of knowledge and progress on the one hand (for example, Hegel) and scepticism about such possibilities on the other (Nietzsche). Indeed, both ends of the pendulum are often included in the approach of a single theorist (Marcuse). While at the moment, the swing would seem to be favouring scepticism, history gives us no confidence in the belief that the pendulum will stay there.

Moreover, I would question the assumption that acceptance of the postmodernist position sounds the death knell for social theorising. Such an assumption is based on the assertion that, following postmodernism, no social theory (presumably not even postmodernism) can pretend to a privileged understanding of the social world. Postmodernism's claims to have undermined the metanarratives of social theory are redolent of Wittgenstein's claim (in very different intellectual circumstances) at the end of his *Tractatus*:

> My propositions serve as elucidations in the following way: anyone who understands me eventually recognizes them as nonsensical, when he has used them – as steps – to climb up beyond them. (He must, so to speak, throw away the ladder after he has climbed up it.)
>
> (1961 [1921]: 6.54)

If absolute uncertainty and relativism are accepted, there is little else for the social theorist to say, for what she says can claim no superiority in terms of adequacy over that which anyone else says. However, a brief perusal of publishers' lists will quickly disabuse the reader of the idea that postmodernists are prepared to accept Wittgenstein's final piece of advice that 'what we cannot speak about we must pass over in silence' (1961: 7). Despite their epistemological modesty, postmodernists certainly have a lot to say for themselves.

All in all, I think the signs are that social theory is in little danger of demise. Indeed, it is my personal hope that it will continue to thrive, not least by breaking out of the ivory tower of esoteric discourse to which it has so often confined itself. To return to the quotation from Margaret Archer that started this book, 'social theory has to be useful and useable; it is not an end in itself' (1995: 135) This has been the purpose of this book – to be a useful and useable guide to theoretical explanations of that particular area of the social world which is called nursing practice. I can only hope that it has gone some way towards fulfilling that purpose.

References

Althusser L and Balibar E (1970) *Reading Capital*. New Left Books, London.

Andreski S (1974) *The Essential Comte*. Croom Helm, London.

Archer M (1995) *Realist Social Theory: The Morphogenetic Approach*. Cambridge University Press, Cambridge.

Armstrong D (1983) The fabrication of nurse–patient relationships. *Social Science and Medicine* 17: 457–60.

Atkinson J M (1971) Societal reactions to suicide: the role of coroners' definitions. In Cohen S (ed.) *Images of Deviance*. Penguin, Harmondsworth, pp. 165–91.

Bacon F (1868) *The Advancement of Learning*. Oxford University Press, London.

Barber B (1963) Some problems with the sociology of professions. *Daedalus* 92: 669–88.

Barrett M (1980) *Women's Oppression Today: Problems in Marxist Feminist Analysis*. Verso, London.

Beck U (1992) *Risk Society: Towards a New Modernity*. Sage, London.

Becker H (1963) *Outsiders: Studies in the Sociology of Deviance*. Free Press, New York.

Benner P (1984) *From Novice to Expert: Excellence and Power in Clinical Nursing*. Addison-Wesley, Menlo Park, CA.

Benner P, Tanner C and Chesla C (1992) From beginner to expert: gaining a differentiated clinical world in critical care nursing. *Advances in Nursing Science* 14(2): 13–28.

Benson D and Hughes J (1983) *The Perspective of Ethnomethodology*. Longman, London.

Berger P and Luckmann T (1967) *The Social Construction of Everyday Life: A Treatise in the Sociology of Knowledge*. Penguin, Harmondsworth.

Berlant J (1975) *Profession and Monopoly*. University of California Press, Berkeley, CA.

Bhaskar R (1978) *A Realist Theory of Science*, 2nd edn, Harvester, Hassocks.

Bhaskar R (1989a) *A Philosophical Critique of the Contemporary Human Sciences*. Harvester Wheatsheaf, Hemel Hempstead.

Bhaskar R (1989b) *Reclaiming Reality: A Critical Introduction to Contemporary Philosophy*. Verso, London.

Bloor M and McIntosh J (1990) Surveillance and concealment: a comparison of techniques of client resistance in therapeutic communities and health visiting. In Burley S and McKegany N (eds) *Readings in Medical Sociology*. Routledge, London, pp. 159–81.

Blumer H (1962) Society as symbolic interaction. In Rose A (ed.) *Human Behavior and Social Processes: An Interactionist Approach*. Routledge & Kegan Paul, London, pp. 179–92.

Blumer H (1966) Sociological implications of the thought of George Herbert Mead. *American Journal of Sociology* 71: 535–48.

Blumer H (1969) *Symbolic Interactionism: Perspective and Method*. Prentice Hall, Englewood Cliffs, NJ.

Bologh R (1990) *Love or Greatness: Max Weber and Masculine Thinking – a Feminist Enquiry*. Unwin Hyman, London.

Bottomore T (1984) *The Frankfurt School*. Ellis Horwood/Tavistock, London.

Bottomore T and Rubel M (1963) *Karl Marx: Selected Writings in Sociology and Social Philosophy*. Penguin, Harmondsworth.

Bowers L (1992a) Ethnomethodology I: an approach to nursing research. *International Journal of Nursing Studies* 29: 59–67.

Bowers L (1992b) Ethnomethodology II: a study of the community psychiatric nurse in the patient's home. *International Journal of Nursing Studies* 29: 69–79.

Bridges J and Lynam J (1993) Informal carers: a Marxist analysis of social, political, and economic forces underpinning the role. *Advances in Nursing Science* 15(3): 33–48.

Brown C (1984) *Black and White in Britain*. Heinemann, London.

Bryant C and Jary D (1991) *Giddens' Theory of Structuration: A Critical Appreciation*. Routledge, London.

Campbell R and Porter S (1997) Feminist theory and the sociology of childbirth: a response to Ellen Annandale and Judith Clark. *Sociology of Health and Illness* 19(3): 348–58.

Carlson R (1996) The political economy of AIDS among drug users in the United States: beyond blaming the victim or powerful others. *American Anthropologist* 98: 266–78.

Carr-Saunders A and Wilson P (1933) *The Professions*. Oxford University Press, London.

Cartwright A and O'Brien M (1976) Social class variations in health care and in the nature of general practitioner consultations. In Stacey M (ed.) *The Sociology of the NHS*, Sociological Review Monograph No. 22, London.

Cheek J and Porter S (1997) Reviewing Foucault: possibilities and problems for nursing and health care. *Nursing Inquiry* 4: 108–19.

Cheek J and Rudge T (1994) Inquiry into nursing as textually mediated discourse. In Chinn P (ed.) *Advances in Methods of Inquiry for Nursing*. Aspen, Gaithersburg.

Chetley A (1990) *Healthy Business: World Health and the Pharmaceutical Industry*. Routledge, London.

Chetley A (1995) Pill pushers, drug dealers. *New Internationalist* 272: 22–3.

Cohen P (1968) *Modern Social Theory*. Heinemann, London.

Collier A (1994) *Critical Realism: An Introduction to Roy Bhaskar's Philosophy*. Verso, London.

Cooke H (1993a) Why teach sociology? *Nurse Education Today* **13**: 210–16.

Cooke H (1993b) Boundary work in the nursing curriculum: the case of sociology. *Journal of Advanced Nursing* **18**: 1990–98.

Cooley C H (1942) *Social Organization*. Dryden Press, New York.

Craib I (1984) *Modern Social Theory: from Parsons to Habermas*. Wheatsheaf, Brighton.

Craib I (1992) *Anthony Giddens*. Routledge, London.

Craib I (1997) *Classical Social Theory: An Introduction to the Thought of Marx, Weber, Durkheim and Simmel*. Oxford University Press, Oxford.

Crompton R (1987) Gender, status and professionalism. *Sociology* **21**: 413–28.

Daly J (1996) *Marx: Justice and Dialectic*. Greenwich Exchange, Belfast.

Davies C (1995) *Gender and the Professional Predicament in Nursing*. Open University Press, Buckingham.

Department of Health (1993) *Changing Childbirth. Part I. Report of the Expert Maternity Group*. HMSO, London.

Department of Health and Social Services (1980) *Inequalities of Health: Report of a Research Working Group* (Chairperson: Sir Douglas Black). DHSS, London.

Dingwall R, Rafferty A M and Webster C (1988) *An Introduction to the Social History of Nursing*. Routledge, London.

Doyal L (1979) *The Political Economy of Health*. Pluto, London.

Dryfoos J (1991) Preventing high-risk behavior. *American Journal of Public Health* **81**: 157–8.

Durkheim E (1938) *The Rules of Sociological Method*. Free Press, New York.

Durkheim E (1951) *Suicide*. Free Press, New York.

Durkheim E (1964) *The Division of Labour in Society*. Free Press, New York.

Engels F (1973) *The Condition of the Working Class in England*. Progress Publishers, Moscow.

Engels F (1985) *The Origin of the Family, Private Property, and the State*. Penguin, Harmondsworth.

Evans J (1995) *Feminist Theory Today: An Introduction to Second-Wave Feminism*. Sage, London.

Evans M (1997) *Introducing Contemporary Feminist Thought*. Polity Press, Cambridge.

Fanon F (1978) Medicine and colonialism. In Ehrenreich J (ed.) *The Cultural Crisis of Modern Medicine*. Monthly Review Press, New York, pp. 229–51.

Few C (1997) The politics of sex research and constructions of female sexuality: what relevance to sexual health work with young women? *Journal of Advanced Nursing* **25**: 615–25.

Firestone S (1979) *The Dialectic of Sex: The Case for Feminist Revolution*. Women's Press, London.

Flexner A (1915) Is social work a profession? In *Proceedings of the National Conference of Charities and Correction*. Hildman, Chicago.

Foucault M (1970) *The Order of Things: An Archaeology of the Human Sciences*. Random House, New York.

Foucault M (1974) *The Archaeology of Knowledge*. Tavistock, London.

Foucault M (1976) *The Birth of the Clinic: An Archaeology of Medical Perception*. Tavistock, London.

Foucault M (1977) *Discipline and Punish: The Birth of the Prison*. Pantheon, New York.

Foucault M (1979) *The History of Sexuality*, Vol. I: *An Introduction*. Allen Lane, London.

Foucault M (1980) *Herculine Barbin: Being the Recently Discovered Memoirs of a Nineteenth Century Hermaphrodite*. Pantheon, New York.

Foucault M (1982) Afterword: the subject and power. In Dreyfus H and Rabinow P (eds) *Michel Foucault: Beyond Structuralism and Hermeneutics*. University of Chicago Press, Chicago, pp. 208–26.

Foucault M (1991) Nietzsche, genealogy, history. In Rabinow P (ed.) *The Foucault Reader*. Penguin, Harmondsworth.

Fox N (1993) *Postmodernism, Sociology and Health*. Open University Press, Buckingham.

Friedan B (1963) *The Feminine Mystique*. Norton, New York.

Freidson E (1970) *Profession of Medicine: A Study of the Sociology of Applied Knowledge*. Harper & Row, New York.

Gadamer H-G (1975) *Truth and Method*. Sheed & Ward, London.

Garfinkel H (1984 [1967]) *Studies in Ethnomethodology*. Polity Press, Cambridge.

Gerhardt U (1987) Parsons, role theory, and health interaction. In Scambler G (ed.) *Sociological Theory and Medical Sociology*. Tavistock, London, pp. 110–33.

Giddens A (ed.) (1974) *Positivism and Sociology*. Heinemann, New York.

Giddens A (1976) *New Rules of Sociological Method*. Hutchinson, London.

Giddens A (1978) *Durkheim*. Fontana, London.

Giddens A (1979) *Central Problems in Social Theory: Action, Structure and Contradiction in Social Analysis*. Macmillan, London.

Giddens A (1982) *Profiles and Critiques in Social Theory*. Macmillan, London.

Giddens A (1984) *The Constitution of Society*. Polity Press, Cambridge.

Gilligan C (1982) *In a Different Voice: Psychological Theory and Women's Development*. Harvard University Press, London.

Goffman E (1964) *Behavior in Public Places*. Free Press, New York.

Goffman E (1968a [1961]) *Asylums: Essays on the Social Situation of Mental Patients and Other Inmates*. Penguin, Harmondsworth.

Goffman E (1968b [1963]) *Stigma: Notes on the Management of Spoiled Identity*. Penguin, Harmondsworth.

Goffman E (1969 [1959]) *The Presentation of Self in Everyday Life*. Penguin, Harmondsworth.

Gorman R (1977) *The Dual Vision: Alfred Schutz and the Myth of Phenomenological Sociology*. Routledge & Kegan Paul, London.

Gouldner A (1971) *The Coming Crisis of Western Sociology*. Heinemann, London.

Gove W (1980) Labelling and mental illness: a critique. In Gove W (ed.) *The Labelling of Deviance*. Sage, London, pp. 33–81.

Graham H and Oakley A (1981) Competing ideologies of reproduction: medical and maternal perspectives on pregnancy. In Roberts H (ed.)

Women, Health and Reproduction. Routledge & Kegan Paul, London, pp. 50–74.

Habermas J (1970) Towards a theory of communicative competence. *Inquiry* **13**: 360–75.

Habermas J (1971) *Towards a Rational Society*. Heinemann, London.

Habermas J (1972) *Knowledge and Human Interests*. Heinemann, London.

Habermas J (1984) *The Theory of Communicative Action*, Vol. I: *Reason and the Rationalization of Society*. Heinemann, London.

Habermas J (1987) *The Theory of Communicative Action*, Vol. II: *The Critique of Functionalist Reason*. Polity Press, Cambridge.

Hagell E (1989) Nursing knowledge: women's knowledge. A sociological perspective. *Journal of Advanced Nursing* **14**: 226–33.

Hamilton P (1983) *Talcott Parsons*. Tavistock/Ellis Horwood, London.

Hardon A, Kanji N, Harnmeijer J, Mamdani M and Walt G (1992) *Drugs Policy in Developing Countries*. Zed Press, London.

Hegel G W F (1977 [1807]) *Phenomenology of Spirit*. Oxford University Press, Oxford.

Heidegger M (1962) *Being and Time*. Blackwell, Oxford.

Held D (1980) *Introduction to Critical Theory: Horkheimer to Habermas*. Hutchinson, London.

Heritage J (1984) *Garfinkel and Ethnomethodology*. Polity Press, Cambridge.

Hewison A (1995) Nurses' power in interactions with patients. *Journal of Advanced Nursing* **21**: 75–82.

Hobbes T (1968) *Leviathan*. Penguin, Harmondsworth.

Hochschild A (1983) *The Managed Heart*. University of California Press, California.

Horkheimer M and Adorno T (1978) *The Dialectic of Enlightenment*. Allen Lane, London.

Hughes D (1988) When nurse knows best: some aspects of nurse/doctor interaction in a casualty department. *Sociology of Health and Illness* **10**: 1–22.

Hume D (1969) *A Treatise on Human Nature*. Penguin, Harmondsworth.

Humm M (1992) *Feminisms: A Reader*. Harvester Wheatsheaf, Hemel Hempstead.

Husserl E (1960 [1929]) *Cartesian Meditations*. Nijhoff, The Hague.

Husserl E (1965) *Phenomenology and the Crisis of Philosophy*. Harper & Row, New York.

Husserl E (1970) *Logical Investigations*. Routledge & Kegan Paul, London.

Irigaray L (1985) *Speculum of the Other Woman*. Cornell University Press, Ithica.

Jagger A and Rothenberg P (1984) *Feminist Frameworks*. McGraw-Hill, New York.

Johnson J M (1972) The practical use of rules. In Scott R and Douglas J (eds) *Theoretical Perspectives on Deviance*. Basic Books, New York, pp. 215–48.

Johnson T (1972) *Professions and Power*. Macmillan, London.

Kant I (1907 [1781]) *Critique of Pure Reason*. Macmillan, New York.

Kearney R (1994) *Modern Movements in European Philosophy*, 2nd edn. Manchester University Press, Manchester.

Kermode S and Brown C (1996) The postmodernist hoax and its effects on nursing. *International Journal of Nursing Studies* 4: 375–84.

Leininger M (1981) The phenomenon of caring: importance, research questions and theoretical considerations. In Leininger M (ed.) *Caring: An Essential Human Need*. Slack, Thorofare, NJ, pp. 1–22.

Lister P (1997) The art of nursing in a 'postmodern' context. *Journal of Advanced Nursing* 25: 38–44.

Luckmann T (ed.) (1978) *Phenomenology and Sociology*. Penguin, Harmondsworth.

Lukás G (1971) *History and Class Consciousness: Studies in Marxist Dialectics*. Merlin Press, London.

Lukes S (1973) *Emile Durkheim: A Historical and Critical Study*. Penguin, Harmondsworth.

Lyotard J-F (1984) *The Postmodern Condition: A Report on Knowledge*. Manchester University Press, Manchester.

Lyotard J-F (1993) Answering the question: What is postmodernism? In Docherty T (ed.) *Postmodernism: A Reader*. Harvester Wheatsheaf, Hemel Hempstead, pp. 38–46.

McCarthy T (1984) Translator's introduction. In Habermas J (1984) *The Theory of Communicative Action*, Vol. I: *Reason and the Rationalization of Society*. Heinemann, London.

MacDonald K (1995) *The Sociology of the Professions*. Sage, London.

Mackenzie J and Webb C (1995) Gynopia in nursing practice: the case of urethral catheterization. *Journal of Clinical Nursing* 4: 221–6.

McKeown T (1976) *The Modern Rise of Population*. Edward Arnold, London.

McLaughlin E (1991) Oppositional poverty: the quantitative/qualitative divide and other dichotomies. *Sociological Review* 39: 292–308.

McMurray A (1991) Advocacy for community self-empowerment. *International Nursing Review* 38(1): 19–21.

Maggs C (1983) *The Origins of General Nursing*. Croom Helm, London.

Marcuse H (1961) *Reason and Revolution: Hegel and the Rise of Social Theory*. Beacon, New York.

Marcuse H (1964) *One Dimensional Man*. Routledge & Kegan Paul, London.

Martin Roland J (1985) *Reclaiming a Conversation: The Ideal of the Educated Woman*. Yale University Press, New Haven, CT.

Marx K (1946) *Capital*, Vol. I. George Allen & Unwin, London.

Marx K (1959) *Economic and Philosophic Manuscripts of 1844*. Lawrence & Wishart, London.

Marx K (1970) Preface to a contribution to the critique of political economy. In Fischer E (ed.) *Marx in his Own Words*. Penguin, Harmondsworth.

Marx K (1974) *The Poverty of Philosophy*. Lawrence & Wishart, London.

Marx K and Engels F (1967) *The Communist Manifesto*. Penguin, Harmondsworth.

May C (1992) Individual care? Power and subjectivity in therapeutic relations. *Sociology* **26**: 589–602.

Mead G H (1934) *Mind, Self and Society from the Standpoint of Social Behaviorism.* University of Chicago Press, Chicago.

Mechanic D (1968) *Medical Sociology.* Free Press, New York.

Melrose D (1993) *Bitter Pills: Medicines and the Third World Poor.* Oxfam, Oxford.

Merquior J (1991) *Foucault.* Fontana, London.

Merton R (1968) *Social Theory and Social Structure,* 3rd edn. Free Press, New York.

Millerson G (1964) *The Qualifying Association.* Routledge & Kegan Paul, London.

Mishler E (1984) *The Discourse of Medicine: Dialectics of Medical Interviews.* Ablex, Norwood, NJ.

Mitchell J (1984) *What Is To Be Done About Illness and Health?* Penguin, Harmondsworth.

Morris M (1977) *An Excursion into Creative Sociology.* Blackwell, Oxford.

Morse J, Bottorf J and Hutchinson S (1994) The phenomenology of comfort. *Journal of Advanced Nursing* **20**: 189–95.

Murcott A (1981) On the typification of bad patients. In Atkinson P and Heath C (eds) *Medical Work: Realities and Routines.* Gower, London, pp. 128–40.

Navarro V (1976) *Medicine Under Capitalism.* Prodist, New York.

Nietzsche F (1968) *The Will to Power.* Vintage, New York.

Nietzsche F (1969) *On the Genealogy of Morals.* Vintage, New York.

Nightingale F (1860) *Suggestions for Thought to the Searchers After Religious Truth,* Vol. II. Eyre & Spottiswoode, London.

Nightingale F (1970) *Notes on Nursing: What it Is and What it Is Not.* Duckworth, London.

Parkin F (1979) *Marxism and Class Theory: A Bourgeois Critique.* Tavistock, London.

Parkin F (1982) *Max Weber.* Tavistock/Ellis Horwood, London

Parsons T (1937) *The Structure of Social Action.* McGraw-Hill, New York.

Parsons T (1951) *The Social System.* Free Press, New York.

Paul J (1978) Medicine and imperialism. In Ehrenreich J (ed.) *The Cultural Crisis of Modern Medicine.* Monthly Review Press, New York, pp. 271–86.

Pearson A and Baker B (1992) A comparison of quality care using Phaneuf's nursing audit. *Australian Clinical Review* **12**: 41–8.

Pinch W (1994) Vertical transmission in HIV infection/AIDS: a feminist perspective. *Journal of Advanced Nursing* **19**: 36–44.

Porter S (1991) A participant observation study of power relations between nurses and doctors in a general hospital. *Journal of Advanced Nursing* **16**: 728–35.

Porter S (1992) The poverty of professionalization: a critical analysis of strategies for the occupational advancement of nursing. *Journal of Advanced Nursing* **17**: 720–6.

Porter S (1993) Critical realist ethnography: the case of racism and professionalism in a medical setting. *Sociology* **27**: 591–609.

Porter S (1994) New nursing: the road to freedom? *Journal of Advanced Nursing* **20**: 269–74.

Porter S (1995a) Sociology and the nursing curriculum: a defence. *Journal of Advanced Nursing* **21**: 1130–5.

Porter S (1995b) Northern nursing: the limits of idealism. *Irish Journal of Sociology* **5**: 22–42.

Porter S (1996a) Contra-Foucault: soldiers, nurses and power. *Sociology* **30**: 59–78.

Porter S (1996b) Real bodies, real needs: a critique of the application of Foucault's philosophy to nursing. *Social Sciences in Health* **2**: 218–27.

Prior P (1995) Surviving psychiatric institutionalisation: a case study. *Sociology of Health and Illness* **17**: 651–67.

Purkis M E (1994) Entering the field: intrusions of the social and its exclusion from studies of nursing practice. *International Journal of Nursing Studies* **31**(4): 315–36.

Pusey M (1987) *Jürgen Habermas*. Ellis Horwood/Tavistock, London.

Rabinow P (1991) *The Foucault Reader*. Penguin, Harmondsworth.

Ricoeur P (1966) *Freedom and Nature: The Voluntary and the Involuntary*. Northwestern University Press, Evanston.

Rock P (1979) *The Making of Symbolic Interactionism*. Macmillan, London.

Roper N, Logan W and Tierney A (1985) *The Elements of Nursing*. Churchill Livingstone, Edinburgh.

Rose H (1986) Women's work: women's knowledge. In Mitchell J and Oakley A (eds) *What is Feminism?* Pantheon, New York.

Rueschemeyer D (1964) Doctors and lawyers: a comment on the theory of professions. *Canadian Review of Sociology and Anthropology* **1**: 17–30.

Rylance G (ed.) (1987) *Drugs for Children*. WHO, Copenhagen.

Salvage J (1990) The theory and practice of the 'New Nursing'. *Nursing Times* **86**(4): 42–5.

Saussure F (1974) *Course in General Linguistics*. Fontana, London.

Scambler G (1987) Habermas and the power of medical expertise. In Scambler G (ed.) *Sociological Theory and Medical Sociology*. Tavistock, London, pp. 165–93.

Scheff T (1966) *Being Mentally Ill: A Sociological Theory*. Aldine, Chicago.

Schiebinger L (1989) *The Mind Has No Sex*. Harvard University Press, Cambridge, MA.

Schiller N Glick (1992) What's wrong with this picture? The hegemonic construction of culture in AIDS research in the United States. *Medical Anthropology Quarterly* **6**: 237–54.

Schneir M (1995) *The Vintage Book of Feminism*. Vintage, London.

Schoolman M (1980) *The Imaginary Witness: The Critical Theory of Herbert Marcuse*. Macmillan, London.

Schutz A (1962) *Collected Papers,* Vol. 1. Nijhoff, The Hague.

Schutz A (1966) *Collected Papers,* Vol. 3. Nijhoff, The Hague.

Schutz A (1972) *The Phenomenology of the Social World*. London, Heinemann.

Sharff J (1987) The underground economy of a poor neighborhood. In Mullings L (ed.) *Cities of the United States*. Columbia University Press, New York, pp. 19–50.

Sharp K (1994) Sociology and the nursing curriculum: a note of caution. *Journal of Advanced Nursing* 20: 391–95.

Shaskolsky L (1970) The development of sociological theory: a sociology of knowledge interpretation. In Reynolds L and Reynolds J (eds) *The Sociology of Sociology*. McKay, New York, pp. 6–30.

Singer P (1980) *Marx*. Oxford University Press, Oxford.

Smart B (1988) *Michel Foucault*. Routledge, London.

Sowell T (1986) *Marxism: Philosophy and Economics*. Unwin, London.

Spiegel D, Bloom J, Kraemer H and Gottheil E (1989) Effect of psychosocial treatment on survival of patients with metastatic breast disease. *Lancet* ii(8668): 888–91.

Stockwell F (1972) *The Unpopular Patient*. Royal College of Nursing, London.

Swingewood A (1991) *A Short History of Sociological Thought*, 2nd edn. Macmillan, London.

Sydie R (1987) *Natural Women, Cultured Men: A Feminist Perspective on Sociological Theory*. Methuen, Ontario.

Taylor S and Ashworth C (1987) Durkheim and social realism: an approach to health and illness. In Scambler G (ed.) *Sociological Theory and Medical Sociology*. Tavistock, London, pp. 37–58.

Thompson J (1984) *Studies in the Theory of Ideology*. Polity Press, Oxford.

Titchen A and Binnie A (1992) What am I meant to be doing? Putting practice into theory and back again in new nursing roles. *Journal of Advanced Nursing* 18: 1054–65.

Tong R (1989) *Feminist Thought: An Introduction*. Routledge, London.

Tucker V (1996) Health, medicine and development: a field of cultural struggle. *European Journal of Development Research* 8: 110–28.

Turner B (1987) *Medical Power and Social Knowledge*. Sage, London.

Turner B (1996) *The Body and Society*, 2nd edn. Sage, London.

van der Peet R (1995) *The Nightingale Model of Nursing*. Campion, Edinburgh.

Van Dijk T (1990) The future of the field: discourse analysis in the 1990s. *Text* 10: 133–56.

van Manen M (1990) *Researching Lived Experience: Human Science for Action Sensitive Pedagogy*. Althouse Press, London, Ontario.

Watson J (1979) *The Philosophy and Science of Caring*. Little, Brown, Boston.

Watson J (1985) *Nursing: Human Science or Human Care*. Mosby, St Louis, MO.

Weber M (1930) *The Protestant Ethic and the Spirit of Capitalism*. George Allen & Unwin, London.

Weber M (1964) *The Theory of Social and Economic Organization*. Free Press, New York.

Weber M (1968a) *Economy and Society*, Vol. 1. Bedminster Press, New York.

Weber M (1968b) *Economy and Society*, Vol. 2. Bedminster Press, New York.

Weber M (1970) Class, status and party. In Gerth H and Mills C W (eds) *From Max Weber: Essays in Sociology*. Routledge & Kegan Paul, London, pp. 180–95.

Whitehead M (1988) The Health Divide. In Townsend P, Davidson N and Whitehead M (eds) *Inequalities in Health: The Black Report and The Health Divide*. Pelican, Harmondsworth.

Wittgenstein L (1953) *Philosophical Investigations*. Blackwell, Oxford.

Wittgenstein L (1961) *Tractatus Logico-Philosophicus*. Routledge & Kegan Paul, London.

Witz A (1990) Patriarchy and professions: the gendered politics of occupational closure. *Sociology* 24: 675–90.

Witz A (1992) *Professions and Patriarchy*. Routledge, London.

Wollstonecraft M (1970) *A Vindication of the Rights of Women*. Dent, London.

Wright E O (1985) *Classes*. Verso, London.

Wright E O (ed.) (1989) *The Debate on Classes*. Verso, London.

Zaretsky E (1974) Socialism and feminism, III: Socialist politics and the family. *Socialist Revolution* 4(1): 83–98.

Zaretsky E (1976) *Capitalism, the Family, and Personal Life*. Pluto, London.

Zeitlin I (1973) *Rethinking Sociology: A Critique of Contemporary Theory*. Prentice Hall, Engelwood Cliffs, NJ.

Name Index

Adorno T, 129, 132–4, 145
Althusser L, 126–7
Andreski S, 9, 15, 20
Archer M, 1, 154, 167–70, 229
Aristotle, 9
Armstrong D, 221
Ashworth C, 19, 33
Atkinson J M, 21

Bacon F, 134
Baker B, 216
Balibar E, 127
Barber B, 26
Barrett M, 186
Beck U, 227
Becker H, 90–1, 102, 104
Benner P, 154, 165–7
Benson D, 118, 124
Berger P, 124
Berlant J, 65
Binnie A, 13, 29–30
Black D, 41–2
Bloor M, 204, 222–4
Blumer H, 85, 87–90, 95, 102, 103
Bologh R, 198
Bottomore T, 57, 152
Bowers L, 105, 122–4
Bridges J, 34, 54–7
Brown C, 176, 226
Bryant C, 178

Campbell R, 170
Carlson R, 44–5
Carr-Saunders A, 68
Cartwright A, 47
Cheek J, 204, 213–16, 226
Chetley A, 52, 53
Cohen P, 33
Collier A, 178
Comte A, 9, 15, 20, 109, 135–6, 169
Cooke H, 4, 5, 84
Cooley C H, 86–7, 96
Craib I, 119, 127, 128, 152, 168, 178, 228
Crompton R, 71

Daly J, 206
Davies C, 13, 27–9, 176, 180, 192, 203
Department of Health, 148, 169
Dingwall R, 75
Doyal L, 42, 46–8, 57
Dryfoos J, 44

Durkheim E, 5, 9, 10–12, 14–22, 33, 58, 81, 125–6, 128, 154, 174, 195, 205–7

Engels F, 35, 40–1, 184–5, 186, 206
Evans J, 189, 190
Evans M, 190, 197, 200

Fanon F, 50–1
Few C, 203
Firestone S, 187–8, 196
Flexner A, 68
Foucault M, 204, 209–26
Fox N, 226
Freidson E, 32, 67–9
Friedan B, 183

Gadamer H-G, 228
Garfinkel H, 105, 117–21, 124, 155
Gerhardt U, 33
Giddens A, 33, 100, 128, 154, 155–64, 165, 167–71, 173, 174, 178, 217
Gilligan C, 29, 181, 189–92
Goffman E, 85, 90, 91, 92–100, 104
Gorman R, 124
Gouldner A, 99–100, 120
Gove W, 92
Graham H, 147

Habermas J, 128, 129, 138–9, 141–53, 156, 160, 208, 221
Hagell E, 181, 200–2, 203
Hamilton P, 33
Hardon A, 53
Hegel G W F, 36, 130–1, 228
Heidegger M, 107, 114, 136, 137
Held D, 134, 135
Heritage J, 124
Hewison A, 85, 100–3
Hitler A, 132
Hochschild A, 157
Hobbes T, 13–14, 22, 225
Horkheimer M, 129, 132, 133–5, 145
Hughes D, 175
Hughes J, 118, 124
Hume D, 172
Humm M, 203
Husserl E, 105–9, 112–14, 116, 117, 118, 124, 136, 158, 207–8

Irigaray L, 228

Jagger A, 186
Jary D, 178
Johnson J M, 79

Johnson L, 50
Johnson T, 65–7

Kant I, 130, 131
Kermode S, 226
Kearney R, 106, 107, 137

Leininger M, 189, 201
Lister P, 226
Logan W, 78
Luckmann T, 124
Lukás G, 194–6, 199, 202
Lukes S, 33
Lynam J, 34, 54–7
Lyotard J-F, 204, 207–9, 211

McCarthy T, 145, 153
MacDonald K, 82
McIntosh J, 204, 222–4
Mackenzie J, 203
McKeown T, 19, 47
McLaughlin E, 154
McMurray A, 54
Maggs C, 74
Marcuse H, 129, 132, 135–7, 228
Martin J Roland, 183
Marx K, 5, 6, 9, 10, 17, 34–41, 44,
    47–55, 57, 58, 59, 60, 81, 125, 127,
    131, 132, 138, 144, 151, 157, 164,
    184, 187, 188, 206, 207
May C, 221
Mead G H, 85, 86–7, 88, 89, 90, 138
Mechanic D, 31
Melrose D, 53
Merquior J, 219, 226
Merton R, 33
Millerson G, 68
Mishler E, 146–7, 149
Mitchell J, 42
Morris M, 118
Morse J, 105, 114–17
Murcott A, 32

Navarro V, 47
Nietzsche F, 212, 224, 228
Nightingale F, 20–1, 72, 73, 74

Oakley A, 147
O'Brien M, 47

Parkin F, 69–70, 82
Parsons T, 10, 12, 22–33, 67–8, 176–7
Paul J, 48–50
Pearson A, 216
Pinch W, 181, 192–4
Plato, 9, 108

Porter S, 3–4, 77–80, 82, 149–52,
    170, 175–8, 225, 226
Prior P, 95
Purkis M E, 154, 164–7
Pusey M, 141, 142, 153

Rabinow P, 219
Ricoeur P, 228
Rock P, 103
Roper N, 78
Rose H, 181, 196–200, 201
Rothenberg P, 186
Rubel M, 57
Rudge T, 204, 213–16
Rueschemeyer D, 27
Rylance G, 53

Salvage J, 29, 152
Saussure F, 126, 158
Scambler G, 147–8, 149, 150, 152,
    153, 221
Scheff T, 85, 91–2
Schiebinger L, 197
Schiller N Glick, 43
Schneir M, 203
Schoolman M, 136
Schutz A, 105, 109, 111–14, 117,
    118, 124, 138, 144, 155
Sharf J, 43
Sharp, K, 3
Shaskolsky L, 85
Singer P, 35
Skinner B F, 88
Smart B, 226
Sowell T, 38
Spiegel D, 193
Stalin J, 133, 207
Swingewood A, 121
Sydie R, 18

Taylor S, 19, 33
Thompson J, 144
Tierney A, 78
Titchen A, 13, 29–30
Tong R, 203
Tucker V, 52, 54
Turner B, 31, 227

Van der Peet R, 21
Van Dijk T, 213
Van Manen M, 114

Watson J, 189, 201
Watson J B, 88
Webb C, 203
Weber M, 5, 6, 9, 10, 12, 58–64, 65,
    66, 69, 73, 81, 82, 83, 105, 109–12,

124, 125, 128, 138, 139–41, 142, 148, 195, 206, 219
Whitehead M, 41
Wilson P, 68
Wittgenstein L, 120, 229

Witz A, 59, 70, 71–7, 82, 180
Wollstonecraft M, 182–3
Wright E O, 81

Zaretsky E, 185, 186
Zeitlin I, 100

Subject Index

Accident and emergency departments, 87
AIDS, 43–5, 181, 192–4
alienation, see capitalism
allocative resources, see structuration theory
anomie, 17–20, 23
authoritative resources, see structuration theory

Biomedical model, 2
bracketing, 108, 113
breaching experiment, see ethnomethodology

Capitalism, 5, 34–57, 58–9, 71, 81, 125, 127, 131–7, 138, 139–41, 145, 174, 184–6, 195–6, 199, 206
    and alienation, 39–40, 44, 127, 136–7, 199
    and exploitation, 38–40, 41, 42–3, 71, 81, 132, 136
    and imperialism, 48–52
    private property, 39–40, 184–5
capitalist ideology, see ideology
care of the elderly, 54–7, 100–3
care plans, see nursing process
caring, 28, 48, 57, 61, 181, 189–94, 198–202, 212, 216
case notes, 204, 213–16
child care, 185, 193, 198–9, 222–4
childbirth, 46, 147–8, 150, 169–71, 187–8, 196
    home birth, 169–71
    human reproduction, 46, 187–8, 196
    pregnancy, 147–8, 170
class, 39–42, 45–8, 55–7, 59–64, 66, 70, 71, 73, 80–2, 85, 132–3, 155, 183–7, 195–6, 206, 222, 227
clinical gaze, see surveillance

collective consciousness, 15–17, 19, 22
comfort, 14, 38, 105, 114–17, 149, 205, 206
communicative action, 129, 138–53, 208
communism, 35, 40, 174, 206
community psychiatric nursing, 122–4
critical realism, 6, 10, 128, 154, 171–8, 179, 228
critical theory, 10, 58, 125, 128, 129–53, 156, 179, 197, 201, 208
cultural feminism, see feminisms

Determinism, 27, 36, 88–9, 95, 102, 163, 172
deviance, 90–2
dialectics, 36–7, 39–40, 133, 137, 187–8
discourse analysis, 124, 213
discursive formations, 210–11
documentary method, see ethnomethodology
drug use, 43–5
dual closure, see social closure
duality of structure, see structuration theory

Economism, 174, 186
education, 4, 12, 23, 63–4, 68, 73, 77, 84, 141, 182, 183, 201–2, 222
emergent theory, 15, 174
Enlightenment, 9, 130, 133–5, 141, 179, 181, 182, 189, 205–6, 207, 209
epistemology, 1–2, 108, 194–202
et cetera rule, see ethnomethodology
ethics, 53, 64, 67, 139–41, 145, 189–94, 201, 206
ethnography, 175
ethnomethodology, 5, 83, 105, 117–24
    breaching experiment, 119
    documentary method, 119–20

et cetera rule, 121
indexicality, 121
exploitation, *see* capitalism and gender

Family, 11–12, 18, 21, 23, 25, 56,
    110, 125, 156, 182, 184–5, 188,
    193, 220
feminine mystique, 183
feminisms, 6, 10, 18, 27–9, 71–7, 82,
    145, 178, 179, 180, 181–203
    cultural, 189–94
    liberal, 182–3
    Marxist, 183–6
    postmodernist, 200, 228
    radical, 186–8
    standpoint, 196–203
    Weberian, 71–7, 82
forces of production, *see* production
Frankfurt School, *see* critical theory
functionalism, 11–33, 99

Gender, 6, 13, 27–30, 71, 76, 146,
    157, 176, 181–202, 227
    and exploitation, 71, 184, 198–9
genealogy, 212

Health visiting, 77, 204, 220, 222–4,
    225
historical materialism, 35–40, 137,
    186–7
holistic care, 57, 107–8, 203, 221–2
home birth, *see* childbirth
human reproduction, *see* childbirth

Idealism, 36, 77, 80, 107, 137, 156,
    171
ideology, 3–4, 47–52, 55–7, 127, 131,
    133–6, 154–5, 175–8, 197, 223
    capitalist, 47–52, 55–7, 127, 131,
    133–6
    professional, 154–5, 175–8
imperialism, *see* capitalism
impression management, 96–9
indexicality, *see* ethnomethodology
individualised care, 4, 221–2
individualism, 14, 17, 19, 47, 54, 85,
    205, 207
inequalities in health, 33, 40–3
informal care, 54–7, 221–2
instantiation, *see* structuration theory
iron cage, 140–2, 206, 219

Justice, 143, 191–2, 202, 206

Labelling theory, 85, 90–2, 104

labour, 16–17, 28, 36–40, 43, 46–7,
    55, 71, 73–6, 81, 131, 138–9, 157,
    184–5, 188, 197–200
language, 6–7, 15, 87, 115, 120–1,
    123, 126–7, 138–9, 142–3, 151–2,
    155–6, 158, 165–6, 208, 210,
    213–16
liberal feminism, *see* feminisms
lifeworld, 114, 117, 128, 143–52, 221

Marxist feminism, *see* feminisms
means of production, *see* production
mechanical solidarity, 16–17
medical role, *see* roles
medicine, 4, 13, 26–8, 31–2, 45–52,
    64–9, 70, 72, 73, 75–6, 77, 79–80,
    121, 129, 146–8, 152, 157, 162–3,
    166–7, 169–70, 175–7, 200–3,
    213–16, 220–1
mental illness, 48, 85, 91–5, 159
    residual rules, 91–2
metanarratives, 207, 211, 229
methodology, 2, 12, 20, 58, 151, 200
midwifery, 65, 70, 77, 169–71, 220
modernism, 204–6, 209–12, 225, 228

Naïve realism, 165–6
natural attitude, 108, 112–15
new nursing, 13, 29–30, 108, 129,
    149–52
nursing development units, 150–1
nursing process, 77–80, 151, 122
    care plans, 78–9, 151
nursing role, *see* roles

Obstetrics, 65, 147–8, 169–71
one-dimensional man, 135–6
ontology, 1, 108
open systems, 173
organic solidarity, 16–17, 205

Panopticism, *see* surveillance
pastoral power, *see* surveillance
pattern variables, 24–30, 67–8, 176–7
pharmaceutical industry, 52–4
phenomenological method, *see*
    phenomenology
phenomenology, 5, 10, 58, 82, 83,
    105–17, 118, 124, 125, 131, 136–7,
    144, 155–7, 158, 208, 228
    phenomenological method, 108, 208
positivism, 20–1, 33, 105–8, 109–10,
    112, 118, 120, 134–6, 195, 200,
    207
postmodernism, 6, 178, 180, 204–26,
    228–9

postmodernist feminism, *see* feminisms
power, 14, 16, 17, 28, 30, 33, 44–5,
    48, 52–4, 55–7, 59–62, 64–6,
    69–70, 72–7, 79–80, 81, 82, 85, 92,
    95, 100–3, 120, 121–2, 134, 139,
    141–2, 146–7, 150–2, 157, 162,
    165–7, 169, 174, 175, 178, 187,
    193–4, 202, 204, 209, 212–25, 227,
    229
praxis, 195–6
pregnancy, *see* childbirth
private property, *see* capitalism
production, 36, 37–9, 40, 42–3, 48,
    57, 59, 62, 81, 127, 131, 140,
    185–7, 196, 219
    forces of, 37–8, 40
    means of, 37–9, 40, 57, 59, 81
    relations of, 37–8, 81, 127, 196
professional ideology, *see* ideology
professions, 28–9, 46, 59, 63, 64–78
    registration, 59, 64, 65, 70, 71,
    72–8
progress, 130, 179–80, 205–8, 211,
    224–5, 227, 228
prostitution, 184
Protestantism, 18–19, 139–41, 206
psychiatry, 50–1, 91, 93–5, 97, 219
psychology, 15, 86–7, 88–9, 91, 107,
    132, 173, 189–92, 193
purposive-rational action, *see* rationality

Racism, 44, 120, 154, 174, 175–8
radical feminism, *see* feminisms
rationality, 14, 58, 107, 130, 135,
    139–48, 152, 176, 179, 182–3, 184,
    197–200, 202, 205, 208–9
    purposive, 139–48, 152, 179
    value, 139–45, 152
reflexivity, 86, 115, 119–120, 121,
    155–7, 159
registration, *see* professions
relations of production, *see* production
relativism, 208, 229
residual rules, *see* mental illness
roles, 11–13, 17, 21, 23–33, 34,
    46–51, 54, 67–8, 79, 92, 96, 101,
    113, 116, 119, 133, 145, 176–7,
    180, 183, 188–9, 202, 216, 222
    medical, 13, 25–8, 67–8
    nursing, 13, 21, 28–30, 79
    sick, 13, 31–2

Science, 12, 20–1, 26, 35–6, 48,
    105–7, 111–14, 116, 118, 125, 127,
    133, 134–6, 137, 141, 170, 171,

173–4, 189, 194–5, 197–203, 205,
    207, 208, 209–11, 214–16, 219,
    224
self, 29, 86–7, 90, 92–4, 96–7, 100,
    127–8, 130, 194, 198, 208, 211
sick role, *see* roles
social action, 6, 24, 83, 85, 90,
    109–112, 125, 154–7, 160–4, 166,
    167–71, 173–4
social closure, 59, 63–80
    dual, 69–70, 72–7, 79, 80
    as exclusion, 69–70, 71, 72–3, 78
    as usurpation, 69–70, 72, 74–6, 77
social facts, 125–6
socialisation, 15, 22–3, 27, 86
socialism, 40, 42, 132–3, 186, 187
standpoint feminism, *see* feminisms
status, 25, 26–7, 59–64, 67, 69, 70,
    77–9, 82, 92, 93, 151, 157, 177,
    198
stigma, 21, 85, 95–100, 104
strategic action, 143–4, 147
structural conditioning, 168, 169, 171,
    174
structural elaboration, 170–1
structuralism, 5, 11, 83, 84, 126–8,
    154, 157–60, 167–8, 195, 228
structuration theory, 6, 128, 154–5,
    160–71, 174, 178, 179
    allocative resources, 161–2
    authoritative resources, 162
    duality of structure, 163–4, 166
    instantiation, 160–1, 163, 166,
    168–9, 174, 217
suicide, 12, 16, 17–21, 128
surveillance, 204, 218–24
    clinical gaze, 220–1
    panopticism, 218–20
    pastoral power, 221–2
    therapeutic gaze, 222–4

Technocratic consciousness, 141–2,
    145, 147–8, 188
technology, 37–8, 43, 46, 48, 79,
    134–5, 148, 187–8, 197, 205, 220
therapeutic gaze, *see* surveillance
trait theory, 68
tuberculosis, 172–3
urinary tract infections, 209–10
value-rational action, *see* rationality

Verstehen, 109–12, 144

Weberian feminism, *see* feminisms